Frans P.G.M. van der Linden   Development of the Dentition

Development of the Dentition

Frans P.G.M. van der Linden, D.D.S., Ph.D.
Professor and Chairman
Department of Orthodontics
University of Nymegen, The Netherlands
Visiting Scientist
Center for Human Growth and Development
The University of Michigan, Ann Arbor, Michigan

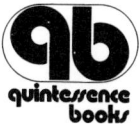

Quintessence Publishing Co., Inc. 1983
Chicago, Berlin, Tokyo, Rio de Janeiro

The author wishes to acknowledge Henry C.M. Reckers and Jos. L.M. van de Kamp for their expertise in preparing the illustrations that appear in this book.

Library of Congress Cataloging in Publication Data

Linden, Frans P.G.M. van der, 1932-
  Development of the dentition.

  Bibliography: p.
  Includes index.
  1. Dentition. I. Title. [DNLM: 1. Dentition.
2. Orthodontics. WU 210 L744d]
QP88.6.L56   1983   612'.311   83-13787
ISBN 0-86715-103-X

© 1983 by Quintessence Publishing Co., Inc., Chicago, Illinois.
All rights reserved.

This book or any part thereof must not be reproduced by any means or in any form without the written permission of the publisher.

Lithography: Industrie- und Presse Klischee, Berlin
Composition: Sharing Sentences, Pacific, MO
Printing and binding: BookCrafters, Inc., Chelsea, MI
Printed in the U.S.A.

Preface

Development of the Dentition is written chiefly to present in a compact, conveniently arranged, and surveyable way the processes that characterize the development of the dentition from the initiation of tooth formation to the complete permanent dentition stage. Extensive use has been made of drawings to allow the reader to grasp quickly and in an easy, accessible form the general aspects and also some particularities of the development of the dentition.
This book is intended primarily for dental students and dentists. For the former it may be useful to receive additional information by means of lectures or seminars in order that they may become familiar with certain facets of the dentition and its development that otherwise may seem strange at first exposure. For dentists, the text and illustrations will speak for themselves, notwithstanding the fact that much information not previously taught in dental schools is included. Further, the dentist will recognize many situations that he encounters in his daily practice.
Development of the Dentition can be useful for those who professionally or otherwise deal with children. This may apply to family and school physicians and pediatricians. No specific knowledge is required to digest the contents of this book. Even the interested layman will be able to gain insight into the interesting and intricate features that characterize the development of the human dentition.

Table of Contents

Preface			5
Introduction			9
Chapter	1	Some Aspects of the Development of the Dentition Before Birth	11
Chapter	2	Development of the Dentition from Birth to the Complete Deciduous Dentition	23
Chapter	3	The Complete Deciduous Dentition	29
Chapter	4	The Emergence of the First Permanent Molars and the Transition of the Incisors—The First Transitional Period	33
Chapter	5	The Dentition in the Intertransitional Period	43
Chapter	6	The Transition of the Posterior Teeth and the Emergence of the Second Permanent Molars—The Second Transitional Period	47
Chapter	7	The Permanent Dentition	55
Chapter	8	Some General Aspects of the Normal Development of the Dentition	59
Chapter	9	Abnormalities in the Dental Arches	71

Table of Contents

Chapter 10	The Development of the Dentition in Class II/1 Malocclusions	81
Chapter 11	The Development of the Dentition in Class II/2 Malocclusions	93
Chapter 12	The Development of the Dentition in Class III Malocclusions	105
Chapter 13	The Development of the Dentition in Open Bites	115
Chapter 14	Subdivisions (Angle), Forced Bites and Deviations in Transverse Dental Arch Relations	121
Chapter 15	Results of Premature Loss of Deciduous Teeth	129
Chapter 16	Factors Influencing the Development of the Dentition	155
Chapter 17	Numerical and Graphical Information Concerning Development of the Dentition	161
Chapter 18	Concluding Remarks	201
References		203
Index		209

Introduction

Learning about the development of the human dentition forms an essential part of a dentist's education. This not only applies to the normal development of the dentition but also to the frequently occurring abnormal ones. To determine in a specific case if the development is or will be abnormal, the fundamentals of normal dentition development have to be known. Therefore those fundamentals have to be taught and will be presented first.
In the supervision and treatment of children, the dentist is confronted with many and often complex features of the development of the dentition. In adults he encounters the ultimate results. These can be understood better in their manifestation and function when one is familiar with the developmental processes involved.
Data and information that are believed not to be essential in acquiring a good insight into the normal and abnormal development of the dentition are omitted here. Primarily this treatise aims to describe the processes that characterize the development of the dentition and to indicate the relations essential in this respect. Numerical and graphical information about a diversity of subjects is concentrated in Chapter 17.
This treatise on the development of the dentition is based in part on data available in the literature and on personal information that the author has received from others. In addition, five important sources have served as inputs: data from the School Study of the Department of Orthodontics from the University of Groningen[12], from the Nymegen Growth Study[81, 104] and from The University of Michigan Elementary and Secondary School Study.[72] Furthermore, the author has been able to observe longitudinally a great number of children. Finally, the author has learned much from the study of prepared child skulls representing various stages in the development of the dentition. This method produced insight into several developmental features that cannot be detected otherwise.[107]
The development of the dentition is closely related to the growth of the face. A treatise describing the former without connecting it with the latter can be considered as incomplete. Nevertheless, for didactic purposes it is preferred not to incorporate in this book the interaction between the development of the dentition and the growth of the face. The author will deal with this subject in a subsequent monograph: *Facial Growth and Facial Orthopedics* (in press).
Finally, the author is pleased to acknowledge the support and assistance received from Dr. H. Boersma.

Chapter 1

Some Aspects of the Development of the Dentition Before Birth

The first local changes leading toward tooth formation occur as early as the sixth week of prenatal life. The oral epithelium in the upper and lower jaws thickens, forming the dental lamina from which local buds arise at each point where a tooth will form.[88] Individual tooth formation proceeds by means of mitotic activity, particularly in the inner enamel epithelium, until the ameloblasts and odontoblasts are differentiated. Predentin and enamel are subsequently formed; the amelodental border is determined.
Teeth are characterized by several typical features. They are composed of the hardest materials found in the human body. This applies particularly to the enamel. The time involved in the formation of enamel and dentin is extremely long in comparison with the formation of other tissues. For example, the calcification of the first permanent molars has already started by the time of birth. When they emerge in the oral cavity at six years of age, their root formation is not yet completed.
Another feature is the almost complete absence of natural repair mechanisms in the enamel and dentin to restore parts lost by decay or trauma. After crown formation is completed, no extension or replacement of enamel beyond mineralization and remineralization can occur. Comparable but less rigid restrictions apply to repair and secondary apposition of dentin.
Moreover, teeth are typical in the feature that their crowns are formed directly at their ultimate sizes. In consequence, their dimensional development runs as if it were ahead of the proportional increase of the surrounding and embedding structures, the jaws. The nonconcordance in increase in size of the forming crowns and that of their surrounding structures lead to several complex and not harmoniously appearing situations characteristic of the development of the dentition. Further, the crowns of the teeth are formed in the region that will contain their roots later. In the adult situation, the roots in the anterior region will require considerably less space than was needed for the crowns during their formation and in their prior-to-emergence period.
A distinct difference exists between the time span involved in the formation of the deciduous teeth and that of the permanent ones. The first deciduous tooth

emerges at about six months of age, the first permanent tooth at about six years of age. Consequently, the mandibular first deciduous incisor has only about one year for its formation and calcification; the first permanent molar has six times as long. The difference in composition between the deciduous and permanent teeth is related to this difference in time available for formation and calcification. Deciduous teeth have a lower calcification level than the permanent ones. Their appearance is more white, hence the term "milk teeth." Permanent teeth are more calcified and become more mineralized, hence they are darker and more yellow in color. The thicker the enamel cap, the more obvious the trait, as demonstrated by the permanent maxillary canines, particularly in males. The relation between calcification level and enamel color is also obvious from the observation that local enamel hypocalcifications show up in permanent teeth as white spots.

Because of the lower level of calcification, deciduous teeth have less resistance to wear than permanent ones. In normal use, deciduous molars soon lose their marked and sharp points and gradually their cusps are worn off. It is not uncommon to encounter exposed dentin in deciduous molars in 10-year-old children, even in Western societies where the feeding pattern induces little enamel wear. A comparable situation occasionally can be encountered in permanent teeth, however, then resulting from the higher calcification level after a considerably longer period of use than is the case for deciduous teeth.

The morphogenesis of incisors, canines, and molars is essentially the same. However, some differences exist in this respect and they have to be understood so that several typical aspects of the development of the dentition become clear.[49]

Forming molars gradually become larger until calcification starts (Figs. 1-1 and 1-2). Thereafter, they continue to increase in size on the basis of interstitial growth of the inner enamel epithelium and because calcification does not start on the different cusp tips at the same time. In a genetically determined sequence, the differentiation of ameloblasts and odontoblasts and the subsequent calcification start on the various cusp tips. Areas not yet calcified maintain their potency to increase in size. When coalescence is attained between the calcified parts of the crown, the distance between two cusps involved cannot increase any more and the intercuspal dimension is fixed. Subsequent formation of enamel still takes place, but it is limited to filling in the region between the two cusps. After coalescence has been completed around the occlusal surface, the size of the crown in mesiodistal and buccolingual directions can increase only by addition of new layers of enamel at the crown circumference (Fig. 1-3).

In contrast with molars, incisors start their calcification only at a single point, at about the center of the future incisal edge. From there, calcification spreads in a more horizontal direction than in molars. The combination of having only one calcification center and spreading in more or less one plane of space—parallel to the future incisal edge—results in a relatively early attainment of a large part of the ultimate mesiodistal crown dimension. This dimension soon can increase only by enamel apposition at the mesial and distal surfaces (Fig. 1-4).

Canines, like incisors, have only one calcification center. Their morphodifferentiation and calcification lag behind that of the incisors and molars. The

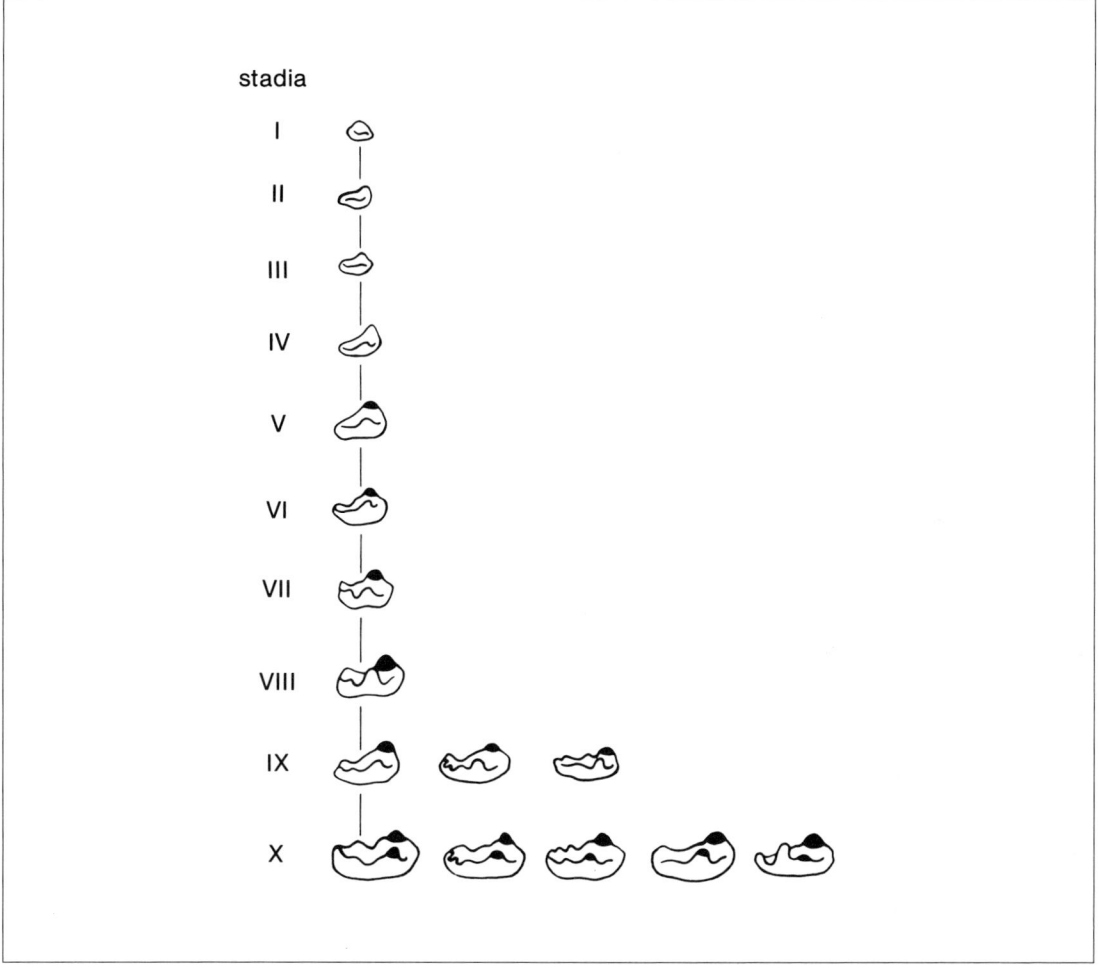

Fig. 1-1 Overview showing the precalcification and early calcification stages of the mandibular first deciduous molar, based on stages in morphodifferentiation. From the first macroscopic indication of tooth development (stage I), growth occurs and morphodifferentiation proceeds. In stage V, calcification starts at one point. The second caldification center does not appear before stage X is reached. The size of the tooth bud crown increases considerably between stages V and X. This increase in intercuspal dimensions continues and does not stop until coalescence between the approaching calcified parts has been realized. Variation in morphodifferentiation occurs after stage IX has been reached, leading to variations in final crown morphology. (Kraus, B.S., and Jordan, R.E. The human dentition before birth. Philadelphia: Lea & Febiger, 1965.)

Development of the Dentition Before Birth

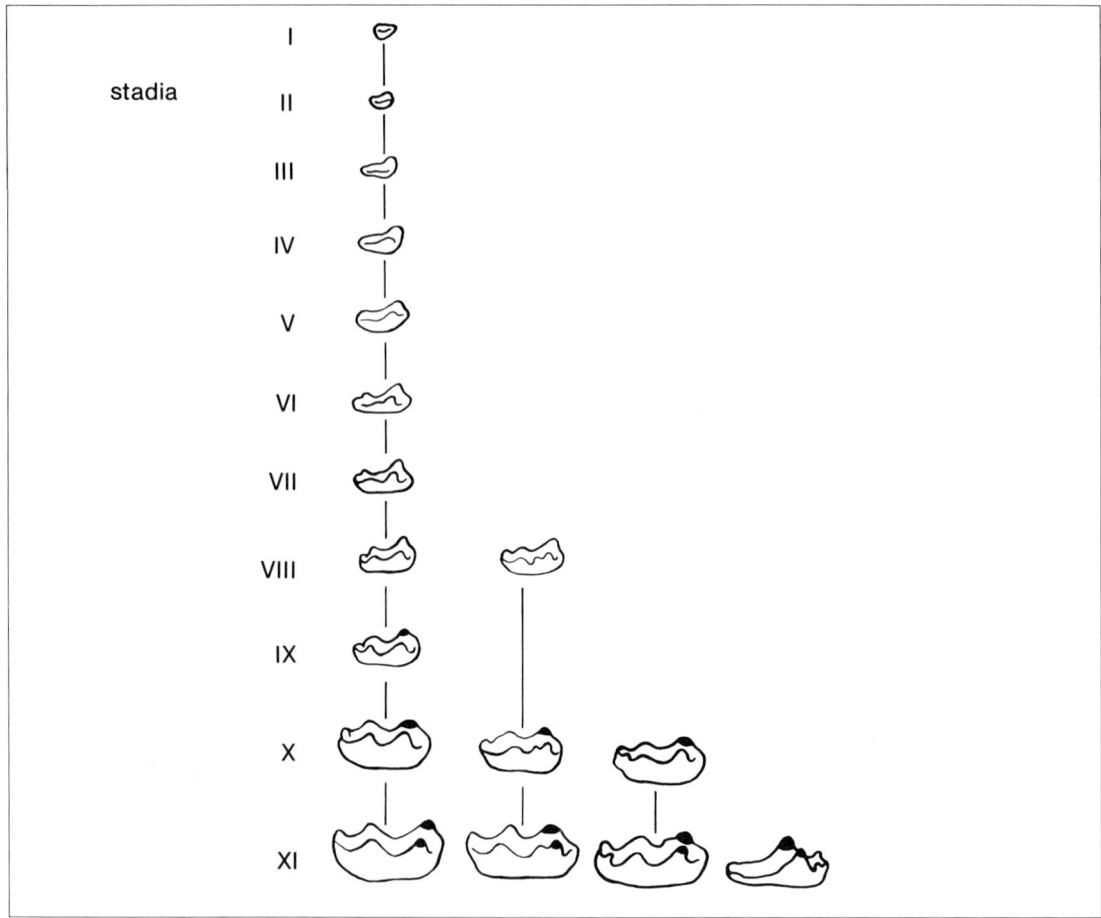

Fig. 1-2 Overview showing the precalcification and early calcification stages of the mandibular second deciduous molar. In comparison with the mandibular first deciduous molar, calcification in the second one starts later. (Kraus, B.S., and Jordan, R.E. The human dentition before birth. Philadelphia: Lea & Febiger, 1965.)

Fig. 1-3 Changes in the morphology, initiation of calcification, and its further continuation in a mandibular left second deciduous molar. Roman numerals are used to indicate the developmental stages distinguished by Kraus and Jordan. All stages are drawn of the same size; increases are thus eliminated. (However, this aspect may well be observed regarding stages I through XI in Fig. 1-2.) Further, morphodifferentiation has proceeded more in the mandibular first deciduous molar than in the second, when the formation of predentin and enamel starts (compare also Fig. 1-1 and 1-2.) The first coalescence occurs in stage XV. The mesial marginal border has been fixed in stage XVI. The distance between the distolingual, the mesiolingual, and the distobuccal cusp tips can still increase in stage XVII. In stage XVIII, the calcification areas have attained coalescence to such an extent that no further increase in intercuspal distance can take place. In stage XIX, the peripherial coalescence has been completed, and in stage XX the total occlusal surface has been calcified. From stage XVIII on, increase in crown size can be achieved only by circumferential enamel deposition. (Drawings derived from illustrations of Kraus, B.S., and Jordan, R.E. The human dentition before birth. Philadelphia: Lea & Febiger, 1965.)

Development of the Dentition Before Birth

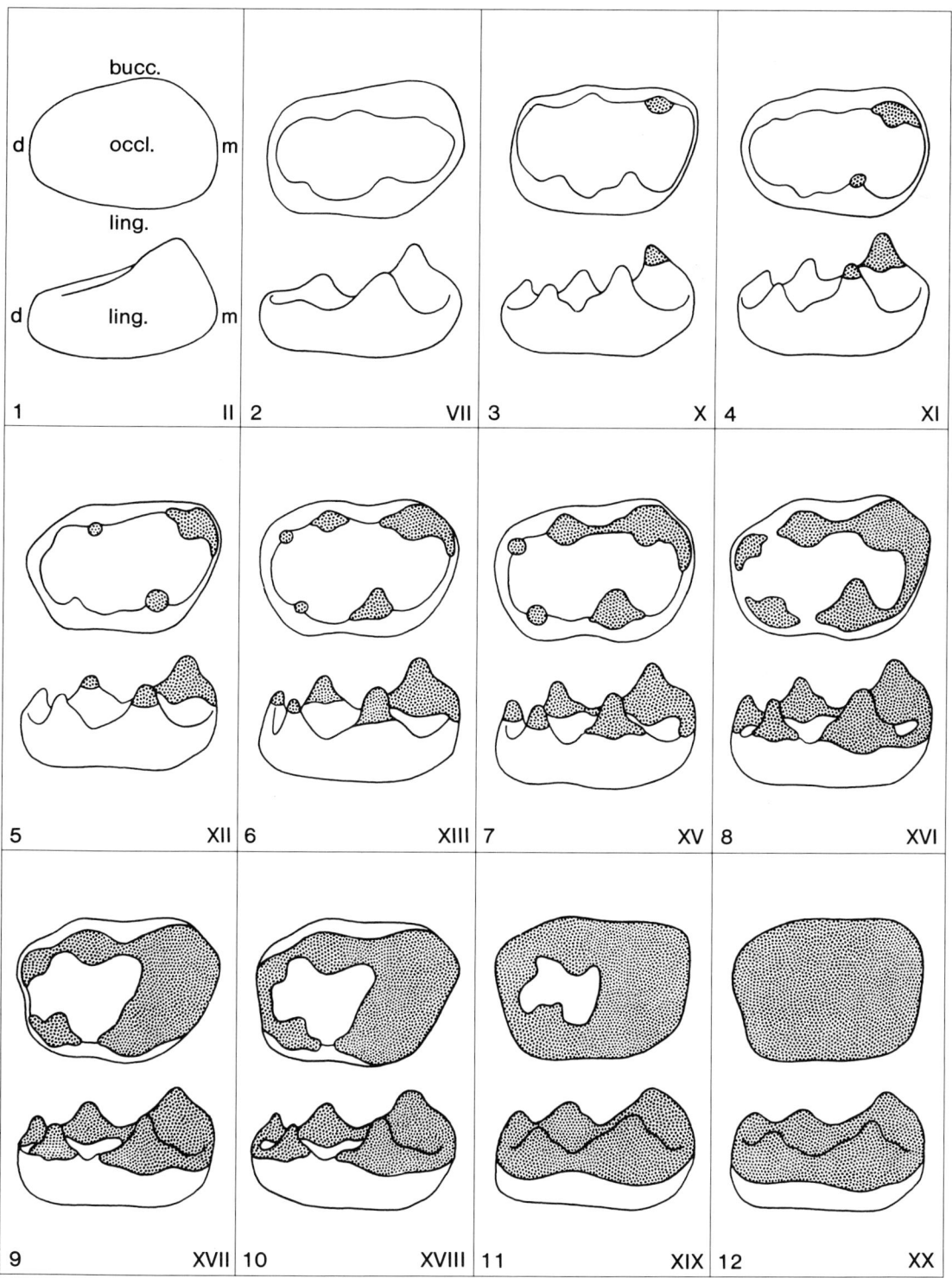

Figure 1-3

Development of the Dentition Before Birth

STAGES IN DEVELOPMENT OF SOME DECIDUOUS TEETH			
wks p.c.	first lower molar	upper canine tooth	upper central incisor
12	dist. ○ mes. 1.0mm 12.5%		dist. ○ mes. 1.2mm 18.5%
16	init. calc. ↓ 2.8 34.5	dist. △ mes. 1.5mm 22.5%	init. calc. ↓ 3.5 54
20	 4.3 53	init. calc. ↓ 2.6 42	 4.5 69
24	init. calc. ↓ 5.8 71	 3.8 61	 5.0 77
28	coalesc. ↓ 6.7 82.5	 5.2 77.5	 5.5 85
32	 7.4 91.5	 5.7 85	 6.0 92.5
36	 7.9 97.5	 6.2 92.5	 6.5 100

Figure 1-4

Fig. 1-4 Development in mesiodistal direction of the crowns of the deciduous mandibular first molar, maxillary canine, and maxillary central incisor. Calcification starts at the incisor slightly prior to that of the first molar and is well established by week 16. At that time, the mesiodistal dimension of the incisor tooth bud is about 3.5 mm, being 54% of its ultimate crown size (see also Fig. 1-5). The corresponding values for the first molar are 2.8 mm and 34.5%. In week 20, the development of the crown of the incisor has proceeded to such an extent that only enamel deposition at the approximal surfaces will add to its mesiodistal crown dimension. In the same week, calcification starts at the canine. The crown size of the molar increases gradually by interstitial growth. Regarding the mesiodistal crown dimensions, values attained at week 20 for the incisor, canine, and first molar are 4.5 mm and 69%, 2.6 mm and 42%, and 4.3 mm and 53%, respectively. In week 24, the second calcification center appears in the first molar; in week 28, coalescence is attained between its mesiobuccal and distobuccal cusps. At that time, the canine has attained its mesial and distal crown extension to the approximal enamel dentin borders. From then on, additional increase in mesiodistal crown dimension can only be achieved by circumferential enamel deposition. The same is true for the deciduous molar at week 32, whereafter crowns of all three teeth can increase in size only gradually and at about the same rate by circumferential enamel deposition.

The incisal edges of an incisor and a canine have only one calcification center; the occlusal surface of a molar has many. An incisor attains a large proportion of its mesiodistal crown dimension rather early because the extension of the calcification occurs in more or less one plane of space, parallel to the future incisal edge. A canine has only one incisal calcification center; however, the direction in which the calcification spreads is at about a 45° angle to the long axis of the future tooth. Thenceforth a canine attains less rapidly than an incisor the stage from which only approximal enamel deposition will contribute to the increase in mesiodistal crown dimension.

The values in mm and percentages of the attained mesiodistal crown dimensions are indicated for the different ages in this figure to illustrate, among other things, that the circumferential enamel deposition forms a proportionally smaller part of the ultimate mesiodistal crown dimension for molars than for incisors and canines. Drawings and data of this figure are derived from Kraus, B.S., and Jordan, R.E. The human dentition before birth. Philadelphia: Lea & Febiger, 1965; and van der Linden, F.P.G.M.; McNamara, Jr., J.A.; and Burdi, A.R. Tooth size and position before birth. J. Dent. Res. 51(1972):71).

calcification proceeds in mesiodistal direction at an angle of about 45° with the long axis of the future tooth. The increase in mesiodistal dimension of the calcifying region of canines is consequently slower than it is for incisors. The combination of these factors results in a difference in timing regarding the initial attainment of the ultimate dimension between the mesial and distal enamel dentin borders. Mandibular deciduous canines and first molars reach that stage in week 28 after conception; central incisors in week 20.

Figure 1-5 serves to clarify graphically the increase in mesiodistal crown dimensions of the deciduous maxillary central incisor, canine, and mandibular first molar explained previously, and to demonstrate that the incisor precedes the other two teeth in this respect. Figure 1-6 illustrates the sequence of initial calcification of the five deciduous teeth in one half of the mandible. This illustration further demonstrates the size proportions of the forming deciduous teeth within one specimen (the stages are illustrated on five different specimens).

As has been explained above, the development of the incisors and canines precedes that of the structures that contain them. This difference in development can serve to explain the overlapping of the incisors and canines before birth. The

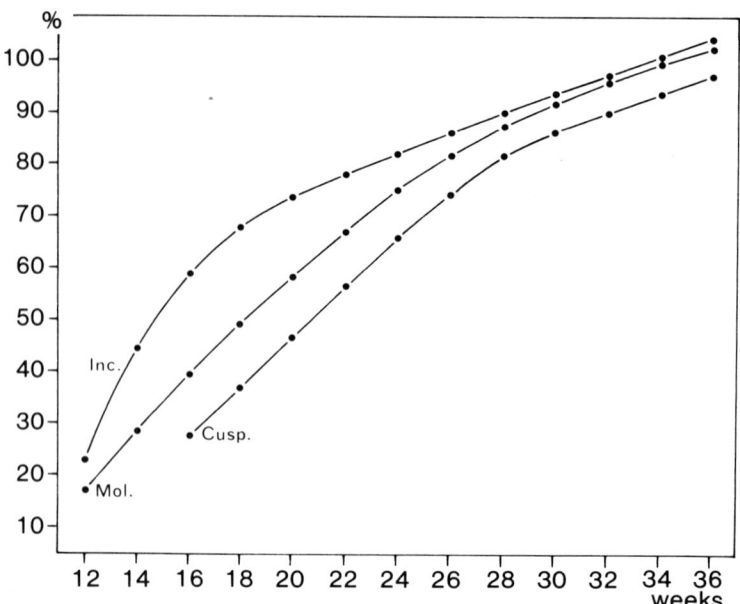

Fig. 1-5 Increase in mesiodistal crown dimensions, expressed in percentages of the ultimate crown sizes of the deciduous mandibular first molar (Mol.), the maxillary canine (Cusp.), and the maxillary central incisor (Inc.). (Based on data of Kraus, B.S., and Jordan, R.E. The human dentition before birth. Philadelphia: Lea & Febiger, 1965; and van der Linden, F.P.G.M.; McNamara, Jr., J.A.; and Burdi, A.R. Tooth size and position before birth. J. Dent. Res. 51(1972): 71.

Fig. 1-6 Sequence of initial calcification of the mandibular right five deciduous teeth. This illustration has been composed of the relevant teeth of five specimens representing increasing levels of development. Calcification starts at the central incisor, followed by the mesiobuccal cusp of the first molar. Subsequently, calcification starts at the lateral incisor, followed by the canine and later the second molar. Calcification is under way at all five teeth before the second calcification center appears in the first molar. The proportional differences in sizes of the tooth buds among the five series are related to the differential increases in dimensions of the deciduous teeth involved.
In judging the five series illustrated in this figure, it must be realized that certain differences in tooth sizes are not related primarily to variations in developmental stages but to variations in tooth sizes that ultimately should have been attained. Teeth that become small are also initially formed in relatively small dimensions. The reverse holds true for large teeth. (Based on figures of Kraus, B.S., and Jordan, R.E. The human dentition before birth. Philadelphia: Lea & Febiger, 1965.)

deciduous incisors and canines are not formed in the orientation that will exist when the teeth have emerged and have attained their position in the dental arch; the spatial conditions do not allow it. "Crowding" of the forming incisors and canines is a typical characteristic of the prenatal development of the deciduous dentition and of the development of the permanent teeth until emergence and sometime thereafter. The term crowding is used to indicate an unfavorable difference between the space needed for a harmonious alignment of the teeth next to each other and the space available for that purpose. Figure 1-7 illustrates the

Development of the Dentition Before Birth

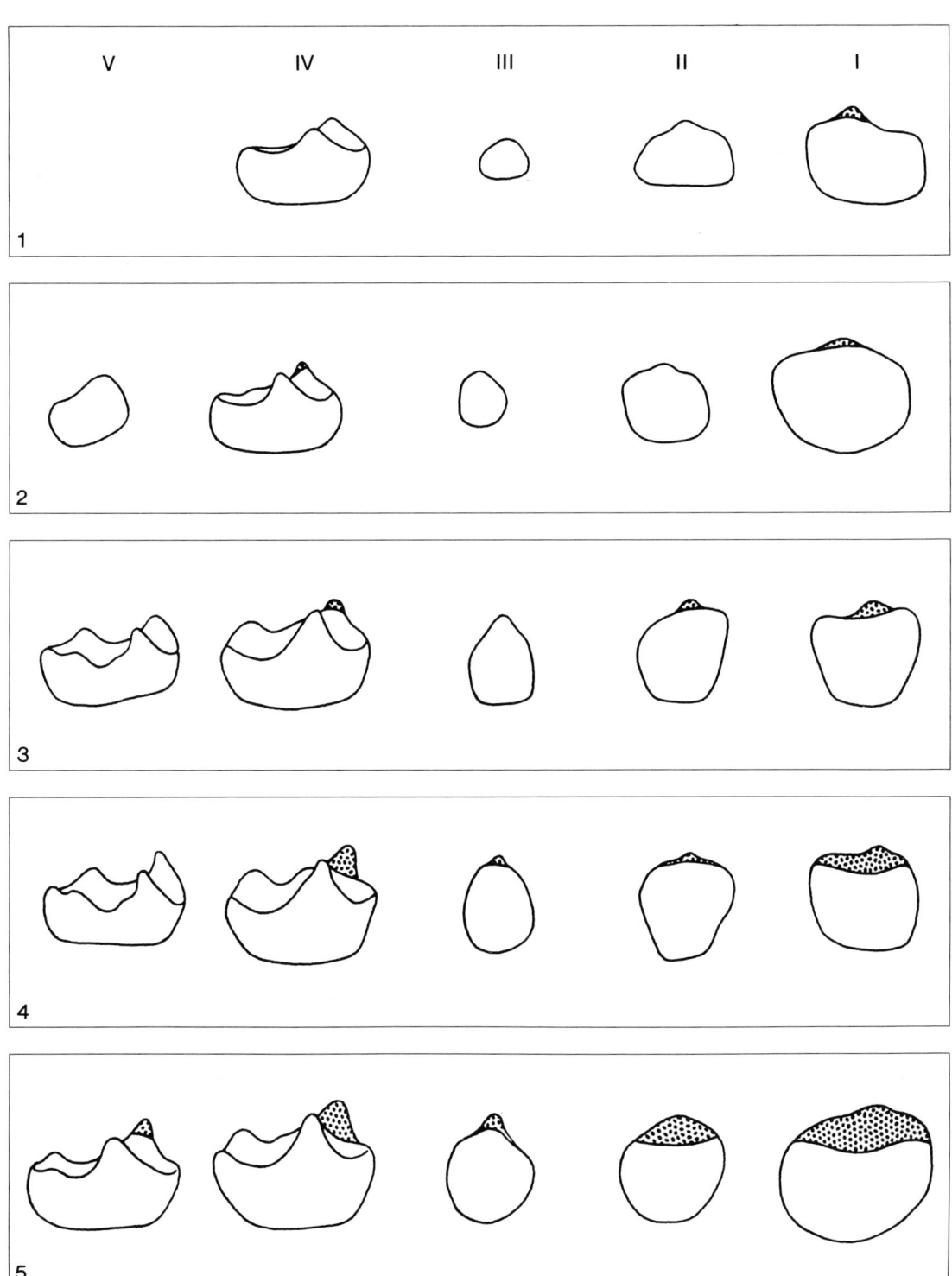

Figure 1-6

19

Development of the Dentition Before Birth

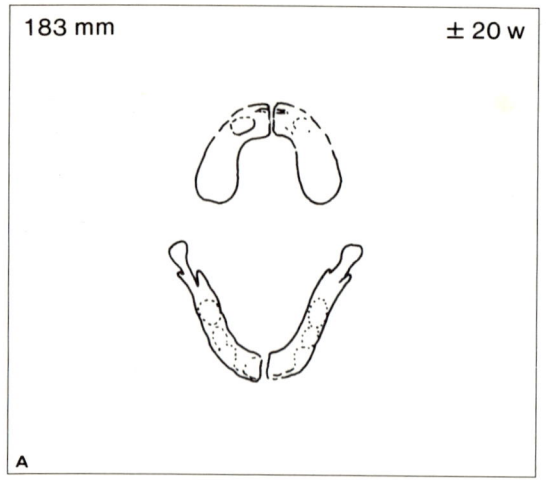

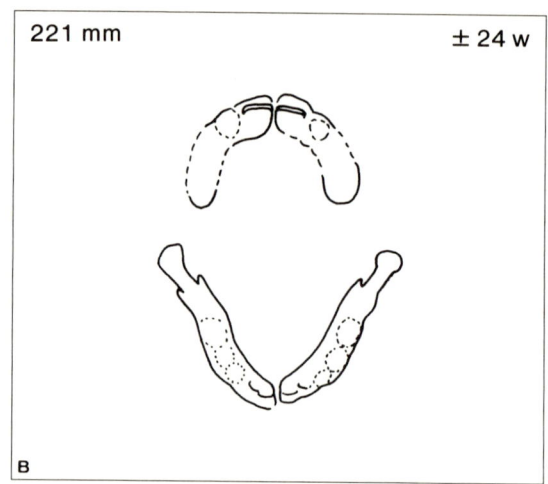

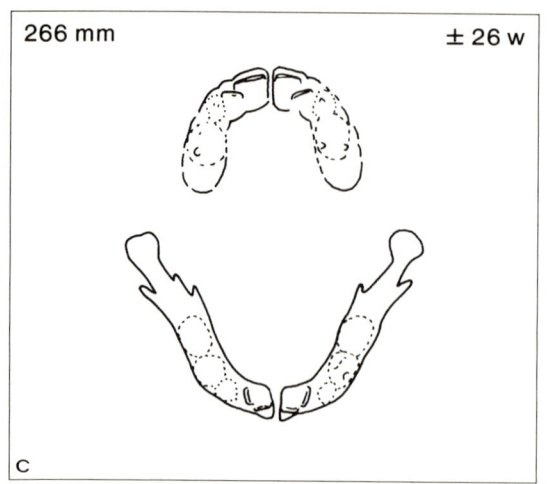

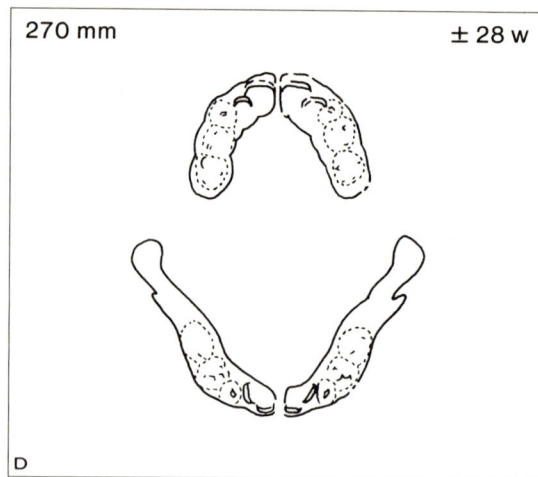

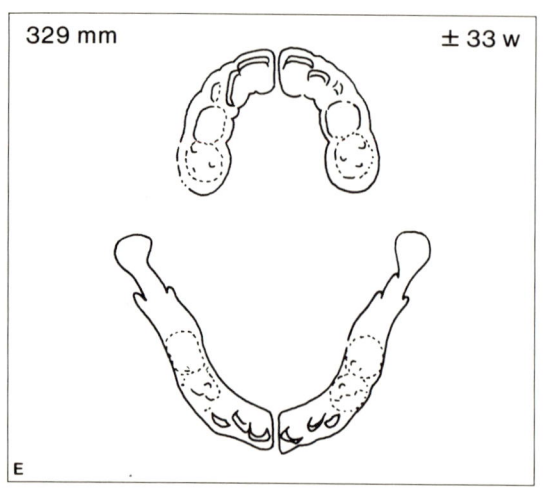

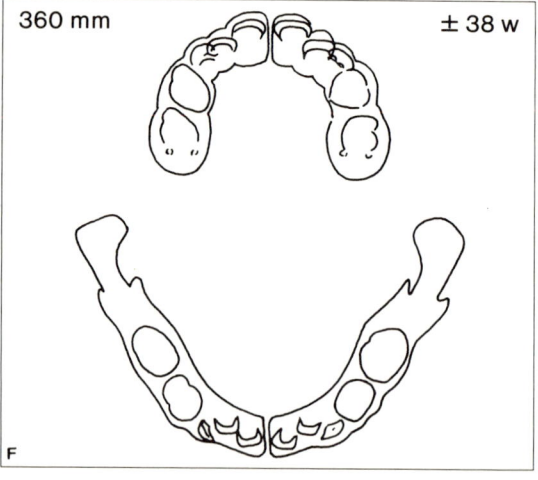

Figure 1-7

Fig. 1-7 Tracings of radiographs of prepared upper and lower jaws of six specimens of different prenatal developmental levels. The mm measurements relate to crown-rump lengths. The estimated postconception ages are indicated in weeks (w).[97]

Here, as well as in Figure 1-6, the limitation applies that preparations of different specimens may show a marked variation in size at corresponding developmental levels, as also would have been the case for the ultimate dimensions had not the development ceased. One child gets larger teeth than another, and the same holds true for the jaw sizes. The dimensions shown in this illustration are not well comparable with each other. Differences associated with the size that ultimately would have been attained interfere with the actual sizes in judging differences in developmental levels.

Further, it should be realized that calcification does not show up on radiographs until a certain amount of radiopaque material has been deposited; calcification starts earlier than can be seen radiographically.

A *Specimen of 183 mm crown-rump length, estimated age 20 weeks. The four mandibular incisors show calcified incisal edges, as do the maxillary central incisors. The crypts (dotted lines) of the other mandibular deciduous teeth could be detected. This was not the case in the upper jaw, as dense maxillary structures were projected over the posterior jaw regions.*

B *Specimen of 221 mm crown-rump length, estimated age 24 weeks. The four mandibular incisors and the two maxillary central ones not only show calcification, they also show mesial and distal enamel deposition. In this specimen too, determination of dental structures in the maxillary posterior regions was not possible. However, the crypts of the maxillary lateral incisors were clearly visible, signs of calcification were not detectable.*

C *Specimen of 226 mm crown-rump length, estimated age 26 weeks. More extensive calcification of the incisors is seen than in A and B. The maxillary lateral incisors are calcified at the incisal edge and approximal surfaces. The mandibular first molars in both jaws show signs of initial calcification. Signs of calcification are apparent at the maxillary canines, too.*

D *Specimen of 270 mm, estimated age 28 weeks. Calcification could be established in all deciduous teeth. The four canines show limited mesiodistal extension of the calcification areas. In all molars, more than one calcification center is present; coalescence seems not to have been attained yet.*

E *Specimen of 329 mm, estimated age 33 weeks. Further extension of calcification at the canines. Partial coalescence at the first molars in both jaws (crypts no longer drawn in; the crown circumference is shown in a dotted line).*

F *Specimen of 360 mm, estimated age 38 weeks (about full term). Large parts of the crowns of the incisors are formed; this is less the case for the canines. The four first molars and the two mandibular second molars show complete calcified occlusal surfaces. No complete coalescence could be seen yet at the maxillary second molars.*

In combination, the six tracings demonstrate the development of the individual teeth and also the differences in developmental levels within the separate specimens. Further, the tracings illustrate the increase in size of those regions of the jaws that contain the developing teeth as well as that of the total mandible. In all six specimens, crowding in the anterior region of both jaws is obvious. The arrangement of the four incisors in each jaw varies considerably. In the molar region, jaw growth seems to proceed at about the same rate as the increase in size of the tooth buds. Overlap of the first and second molars does not occur. In the oldest specimen, extra space is available between the first and second molars.

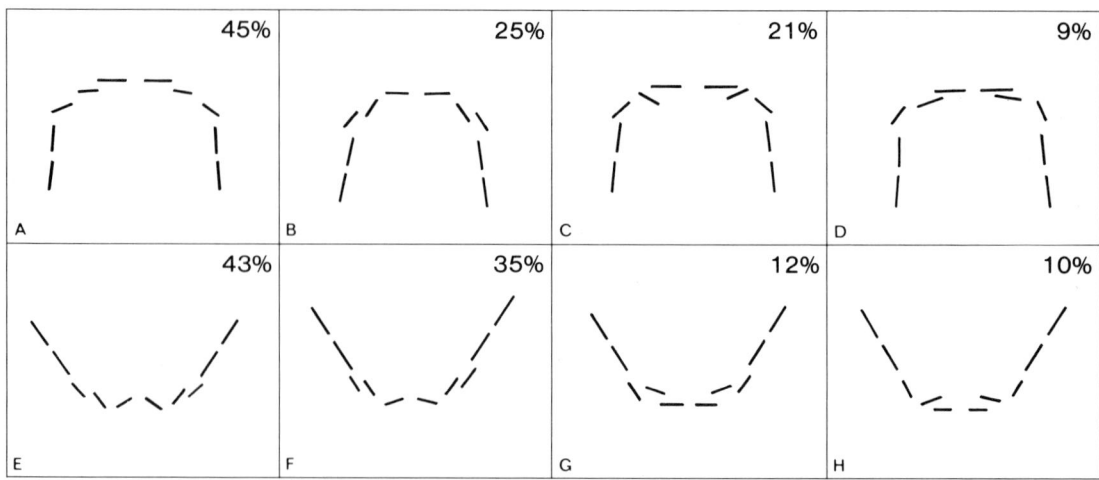

Fig. 1-8 Four different arrangements of the deciduous teeth in both jaws before birth. In the maxilla, the central incisors are always perpendicularly orientated at the median plane. The percentages of observed frequencies are indicated for each arrangement. (Figure and data derived from: van der Linden, F.P.G.M.; McNamara, Jr., J.A.; and Burdi, A.R. Tooth size and position before birth. J. Dent. Res. 51(1972):71).

arrangement of the forming deciduous teeth within the jaws by means of six specimens of different developmental levels. The arrangement is not the same for all six of them. A certain variation is present, as is elaborated in Figure 1-8. The growth before birth of the anterior segments of the two jaws is not larger than the increase in mesiodistal crown dimensions of the containing incisors.[108] Therefore it is assumed that the overlapping of the incisors and canines does not change noticeably before birth, as the extra space needed does not become available then. This will occur during the rapid growth of the jaws in the first six to eight months after birth.

Chapter 2

Development of the Dentition from Birth to the Complete Deciduous Dentition

At birth, the maxilla and mandible are small in comparison with the other structures of the head. Further, the lower jaw is more dorsally positioned in relation to the upper one than will be the case when the deciduous teeth have erupted fully. The regions of both jaws that contain tooth buds grow considerably during the first six to eight months of postnatal life. In addition, a significant ventral development takes place during the first year, leading to an anteroposterior relation between the two dental arches that conforms to the one present in the complete deciduous dentition.[23,24,93,94,101]

The extensive early transverse development of both jaws can be realized mainly because of the presence of the suture in the median plane of the maxilla and of a synchondrosis in the mandible. Both structures are capable of rapid growth. As the synchondrosis in the mandible calcifies at about six months of age, the potency for rapid transversal growth in the lower jaw is eliminated. After a bony union has been established between the two halves of the mandible, the potency of interstitial growth—a typical characteristic of cartilage and not of bone—is lost. In contrast with the situation in the mandible, the maxilla maintains its rapid median growth potency. The maxillary median suture remains until the development of the dentition has been completed. After the occlusion in the posterior region has been established, the transverse development of the two dental arches becomes coordinated. Thereafter the transverse development of the maxilla will be determined mainly by the above indicated limitations in the mandible. As a consequence, the growth potency of the maxillary median suture is only partly utilized, as the mandibular synchondrosis has already been calcified.

The increase in size of both jaws usually is sufficient to provide the space needed for a harmonious arrangement of the deciduous teeth in the dental arches upon their emergence. The crowding initially present in the arrangement of the anterior teeth at birth has disappeared at the time they emerge. Crowding is rarely encountered in the deciduous dental arches. On the contrary, usually an excess of space is available and diastemata are present between all teeth. Sometimes a not fully corrected rotation of an incisor is observed, in spite of the fact that enough space is available for proper alignment.

The development from birth to complete deciduous dentition is presented in Figure 2-1. For an overview of emergence times, mesiodistal crown dimensions, and different stages in crown and root formation, refer to Chapter 17.

From Birth to the Complete Deciduous Dentition

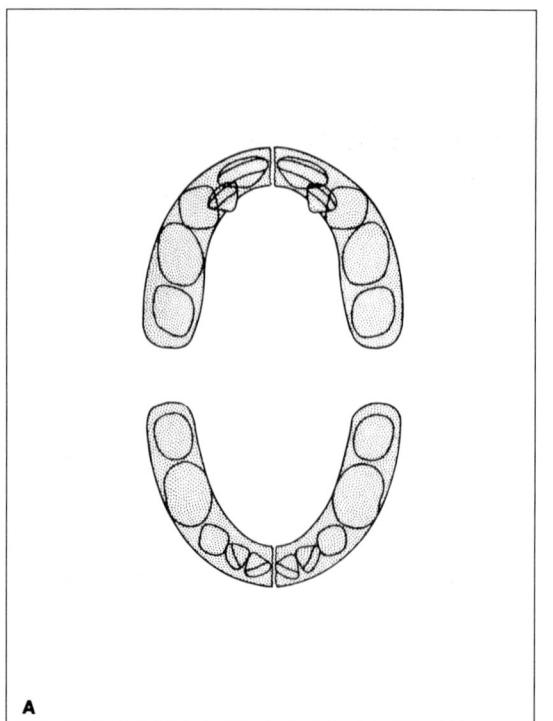

A

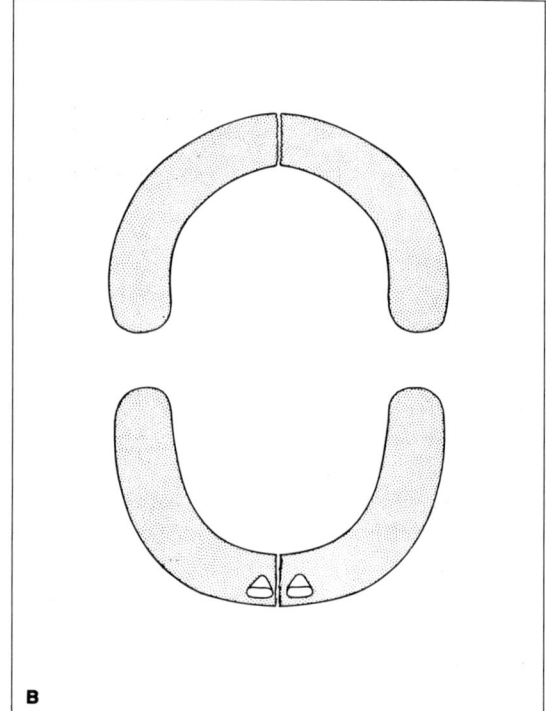

B

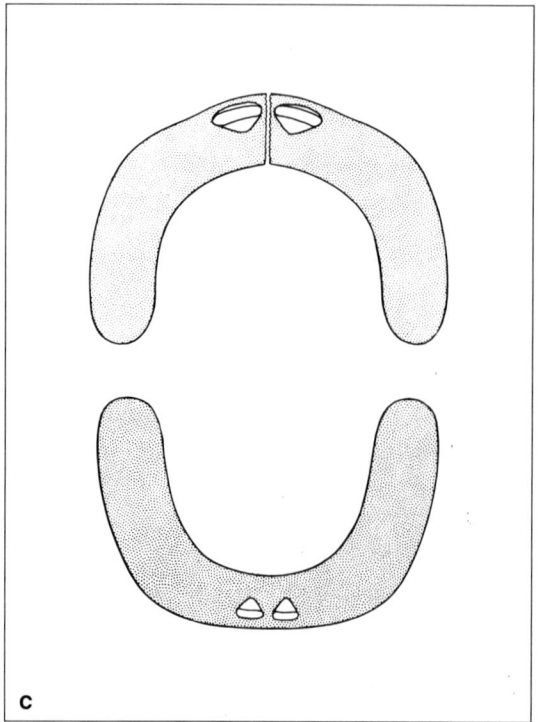

C

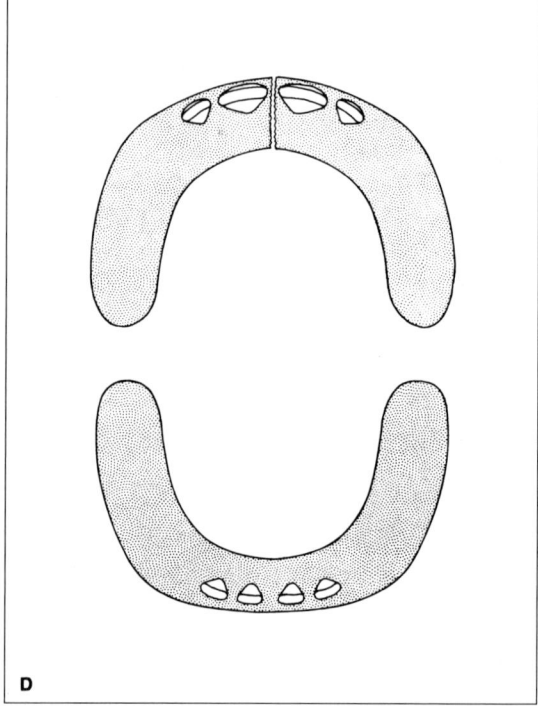

D

From Birth to the Complete Deciduous Dentition

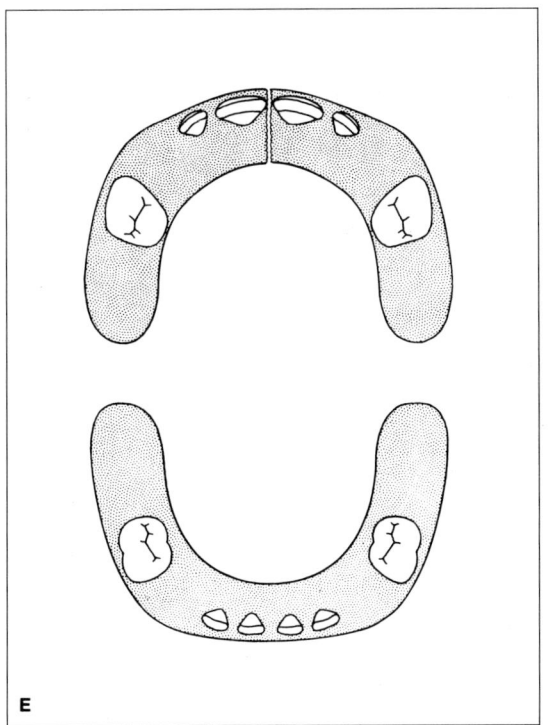

E

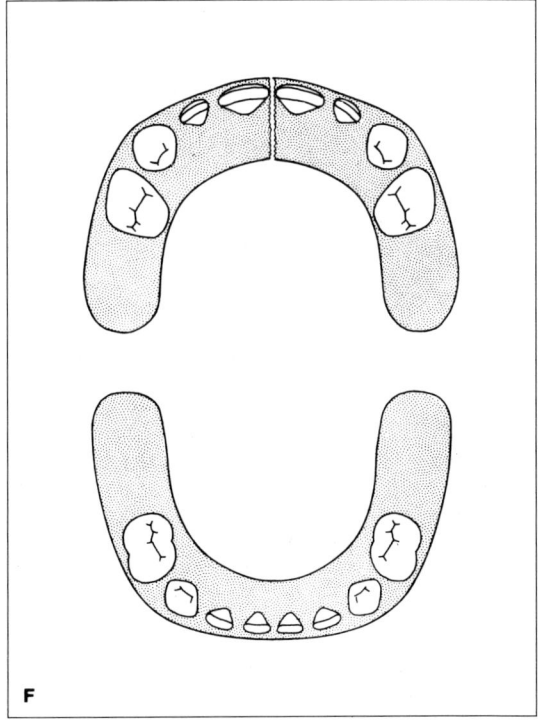

F

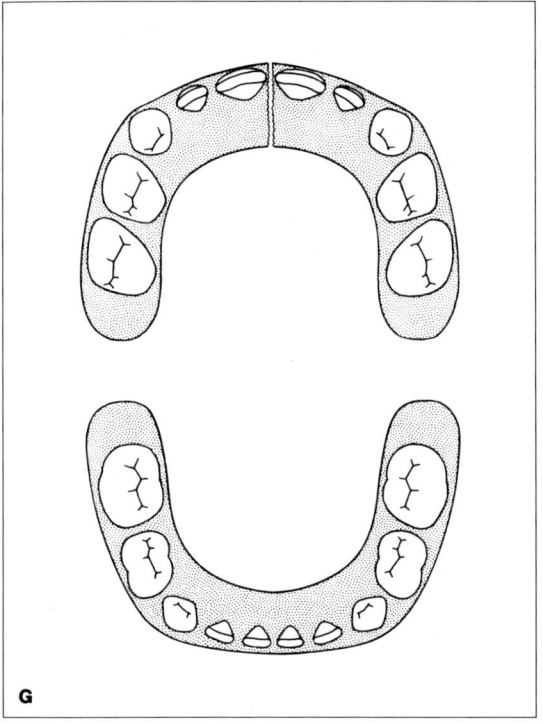

G

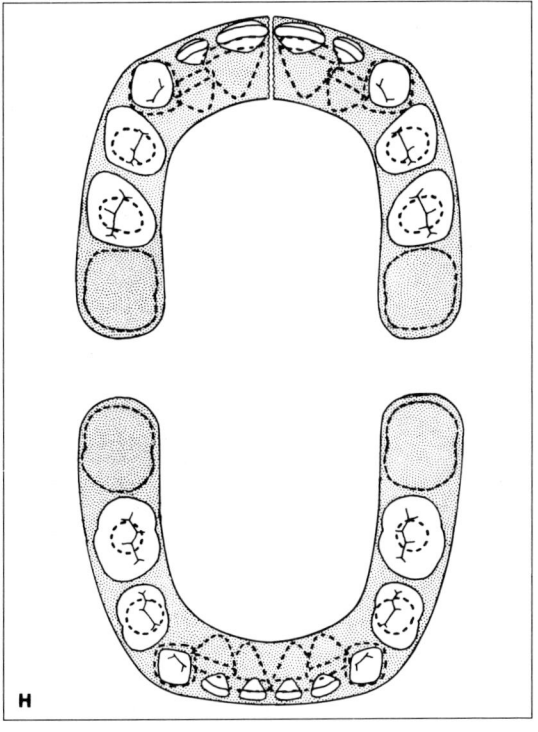

H

Figure 2-1

Fig. 2-1 Survey of the development of the regions in the upper and lower jaw containing the teeth and of the emergence of the deciduous teeth.

A Both jaws are relatively small at birth. The deciduous incisors and canines are in a crowded position. The situation illustrated here is the one most frequently observed. (For variations, see Fig. 1-8.) The deciduous molars are located in the jaws without crowding and often with some space between them. (The already forming permanent incisors and first molars have not been drawn in A through G.)

B From birth to about 6 to 8 months of age, both jaws grow extensively. In addition, a marked ventral development takes place, leading to a more anterior position of the lower jaw in relation to the upper one. The relatively dorsal position of the mandible initially present has changed considerably by the time the incisors emerge. (Only the teeth that have emerged have been drawn.)

C The maxillary central deciduous incisors emerge a few months after the mandibular ones.

D The lateral deciduous incisors emerge at about 1 year of age; the mandibular ones usually precede the maxillary ones.

E After the first year, the transverse and ventral development of the anterior regions of both dental arches and the associated alveolar processes is limited. The posterior regions keep growing. A more or less continuous extension takes place dorsally in the molar region, providing the space needed for the molars to emerge subsequently. The first deciduous molars emerge around 16 months of age, resulting in a vertically supported occlusal contact between the two dental arches. (For the attainment of the proper orientation of the maxillary and mandibular first deciduous molars, refer to Fig. 2-2).

F The maxillary and mandibular deciduous canines emerge in the spaces available for them in the dental arches at about 20 months of age. The changes in position of the previously emerged teeth are limited and the relationship between the two dental arches undergoes little change. Only the mandibular teeth move gradually, somewhat ventrally in relation to the maxillary ones as the anterior development of the mandible slightly exceeds that of the maxilla.

G Finally, the second deciduous molars emerge between 24 and 30 months of age. Their attainment of occlusion conforms to the one described for the first deciduous molars (Fig. 2-2). However, in cases of a close proximity between the first deciduous molars in one dental arch, the already established positions of the former will affect the movements of the latter.

H In this overview of the complete deciduous dentition, the successors and first permanent molars are drawn too. The crowns of the permanent incisors are positioned lingually to the apices of their predecessors. The permanent canine crowns are located immediately above, (or below) the roots of their predecessors, with their crown tips lingual to the apices of the latter. The premolar crowns are located between the roots of the deciduous molars. The premolars have smaller mesiodistal crown dimensions than their predecessors. The reverse applies to the incisors and canines.

The first vertical support associated with *interdigitation*—the interlocking of the maxillary and mandibular posterior teeth*—occurs when the first deciduous molars attain contact (Fig. 2-2). As a rule, those teeth are *not* centered over each other in such a position that no transverse or sagittal translation will be required to reach correct interdigitation. In most instances, the large palatal cusp of the maxillary first deciduous molar arrives with its cone shape within the crater formed by the occlusal anatomy of the mandibular one. The crater will function as a funnel by which both

*In this work incisors are indicated as anterior teeth; all other teeth as posterior teeth.

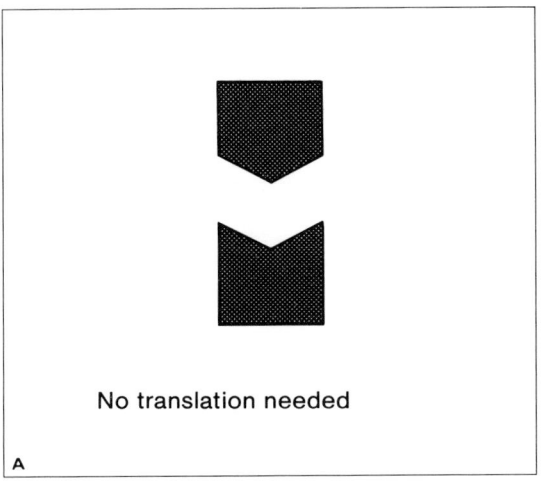

A No translation needed

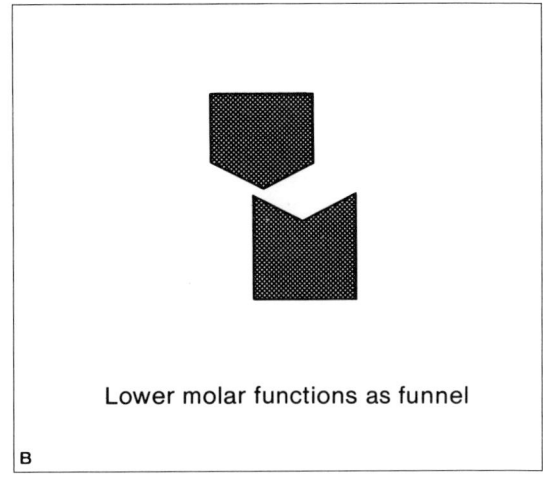

B Lower molar functions as funnel

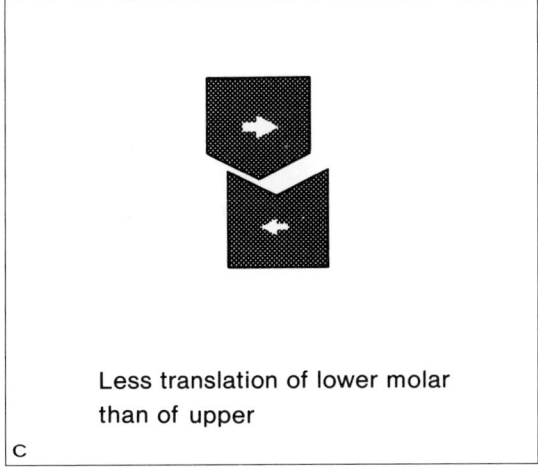

C Less translation of lower molar than of upper

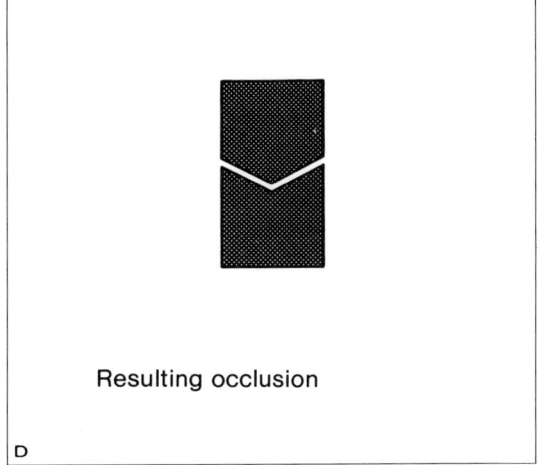

D Resulting occlusion

Fig. 2-2 Displacement of the first deciduous molars in the process of establishing occlusion: the cone-funnel mechanism.

teeth are directed toward each other in the proper position.[89] A required movement of the teeth involved will be derived more from a displacement of the maxillary than of the mandibular molar, as the structures in the mandible favor such a movement less than those in the maxilla. The occlusion in the posterior region is established when the first deciduous molars have settled. Thereafter the relation between the two dental arches will stabilize in the transverse and sagittal direction.

For the position of the deciduous teeth prior to eruption, the relation with the forming permanent teeth, and the localization and formation of the latter, refer to van der Linden and Duterloo.[107]

Chapter 3

The Complete Deciduous Dentition

The deciduous dentition is complete after all second deciduous molars have attained occlusion, usually at around 2.5 years of age. Both dental arches are about half-round in shape. Diastemata are usually present between all teeth and particularly in the anterior region. More than sufficient space is available for a harmonious alignment of the deciduous teeth in both dental arches (Fig. 3-1). In the anterior and posterior regions, the teeth are oriented almost perpendicularly to the occlusal plane (an imaginary plane through the incisal edges of the central incisors and the distal cusps of the last molars). This orientation holds true for the mesiodistal as well as the buccolingual direction. The mandibular teeth occlude slightly lingually with the maxillary ones. The first and second deciduous molars make contact over a large area and function as grinding units in chewing. In occlusion, the mesial surface of the mandibular first deciduous molar is positioned anteriorly to that of the maxillary one; the same holds true for the two opposing second deciduous molars.
The variation in mesiodistal crown dimension of the mandibular second deciduous molar is considerable. In situations with a relatively large mesiodistal crown dimension of a mandibular second molar and otherwise normal circumstances, no mesial step generally is present at the distal surfaces of the opposing second deciduous molars (terminal plane), as is illustrated in Figure 3-1D. The terminal plane of the deciduous dentition will be flush.
Little changes take place in the deciduous dentition from age 2.5 to about age 5. This applies to the position of the individual teeth as well as to the sagittal and transverse relation between the two dental arches. The absence of obvious changes in the position of the deciduous teeth cannot be considered as a sign of arrest in the process of the development of the dentition as a whole. Superiorly and lingually to the deciduous teeth, the formation of their successors continues in the maxilla. A comparable development takes place in the mandible. In addition, the permanent molars are formed posteriorly to the deciduous dental arches. The formation of the perma-

The Complete Deciduous Dentition

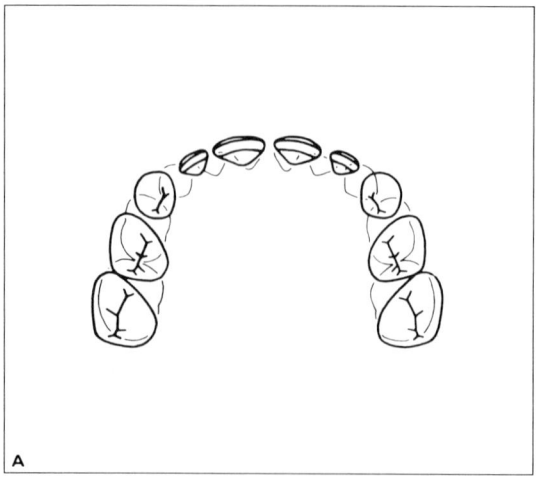
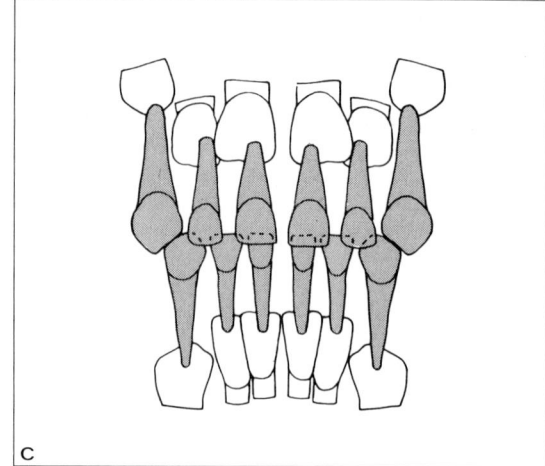
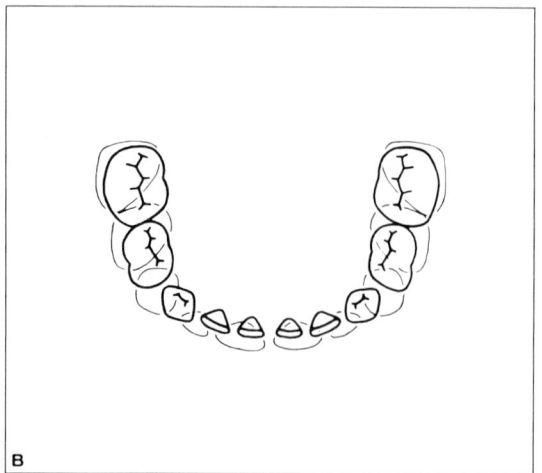
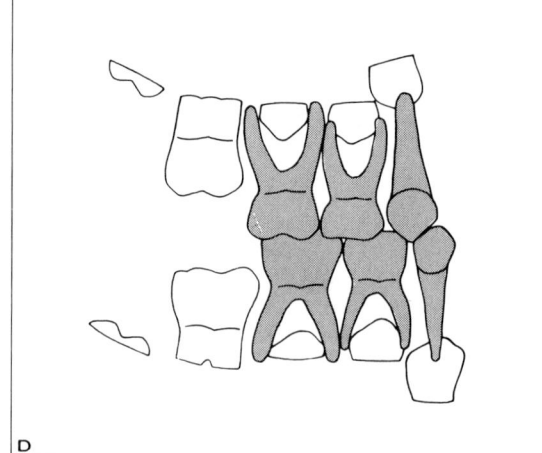

Figure 3-1

nent teeth is a continuous process that takes many years. In both jaws the permanent incisors are located lingually to the roots of their predecessors. Insufficient space is available within the jaws to permit an arrangement without overlapping. As such, the situation is comparable to the one present for the deciduous anterior teeth before birth.

The Complete Deciduous Dentition

Fig. 3-1 Schematic drawing of the normal situation of the complete deciduous dentition. In the anterior (C) and lateral (D) views, the deciduous teeth have been shaded to facilitate interpretation.

A   The maxillary dental arch (heavy lines) presented as it occludes with the mandibular one (thin lines) is about half-round in shape. Frequently, the opposing incisors do not make contact. Often a diastema is present between the adjacent deciduous molars.

B   The mandibular dental arch (now in heavy lines and the maxillary one in thin lines) too is about half-round in shape. All mandibular teeth occlude slightly lingually to the maxillary ones. As in the maxillary dental arch, diastemata are present mesially to the first deciduous molars and often also between the latter and the second deciduous molars.

C   The permanent incisors are located lingually to the roots of their predecessors. The crowns of the maxillary central permanent incisors are located at some distance from each other with the maxillary median suture in between. In the mandible, no comparable median structure is present. The mandibular permanent centrals are in contact with each other or in close proximity. In both jaws, the lateral permanent incisors are located lingually to the central ones. In the maxilla, the incisal edges of the permanent lateral incisors are situated more occlusally than those of the central ones; the reverse situation exists in the mandible.

D   The mandibular deciduous molars occlude slightly mesially to their antagonists. As such, they follow the pattern initiated in the anterior segment, characterized by a relatively more mesial position of a mandibular tooth in comparison with the corresponding maxillary one. This reflects the difference in mesiodistal crown dimensions of the maxillary and mandibular central incisors and, to a lesser extent, of the lateral ones.

The forming permanent canine crowns are located immediately above (or below) the roots of their predecessors, with their crown tips lingual to the apices of the latter.

The forming premolars are located between the roots of their predecessors. The first permanent molars have sufficient space in the jaws. Their roots are already partially formed. The forming crowns of the second permanent molars are located posteriorly to the roots of the first. In each jaw, the forming parts of the permanent teeth in the posterior region with the exception of the canine are at about the same level.

The illustration of the localization of the permanent teeth prior to emergence and their relation to the deciduous teeth, as shown in Figure 3-1 and the accompanying legend, is far from complete. For more information, and particularly for the three-dimensional aspects, refer to the van der Linden and Duterloo Atlas.[107]

Chapter 4

The Emergence of the First Permanent Molars and the Transition of the Incisors— The First Transitional Period

The first emerging tooth of the permanent dentition is usually the mandibular first molar, which appears in the mouth at about six years of age.* The preceding continuous increase in size of the jaw regions posteriorly to the deciduous molars provides the space needed for the addition of the first permanent molars to the dental arches. In both jaws the first permanent molars erupt more or less in a perpendicular orientation to the occlusal plane. This perpendicular orientation exists in the mesiodistal as well as in the buccolingual direction and is in accord with the position of the first permanent molars within the jaws prior to emergence. Frequently the mesial surface of the permanent first molar and the distal surface of the adjacent deciduous second molar are not in close proximity. A diastema between the two teeth present after full eruption of the former can be preserved for a few years.

The anteroposterior relation between two opposing permanent first molars after emergence depends on their positions previously occupied within the jaws, the sagittal relation between the mandible and maxilla, and the ratios of mesiodistal crown dimensions of the mandibular and maxillary deciduous molars. Regarding the latter, a distinct variation exists among individuals, particularly concerning the deciduous second molar. If the mesiodistal crown dimensions of the mandibular and maxillary deciduous second molars are about the same, the sagittal relation between corresponding mesial and distal surfaces will be similar. A mesial shoulder will be present anteriorly at the mesial surfaces and posteriorly at the distal surfaces of the teeth. The terminal plane will have a mesial step (Fig. 4-1A). If the mandibular second deciduous molar is considerably larger in mesiodistal crown dimension than the maxillary one—and this is often the case—then the distal surfaces of the two opposing second molars will lie more or less in one plane. Under these occlusal conditions, a flush terminal plane will be present (Fig. 4-1C). The consequences of the varying forms of terminal planes for the initial contact of the first permanent molars and the resulting occlusion are indicated in Figure 4-1. However, when deciduous molars are

*By *eruption* is meant the movement of a tooth in occlusal direction; by *emergence*, the perforation of the gum tissue and the appearance of the tooth in the oral cavity.

The First Transitional Period

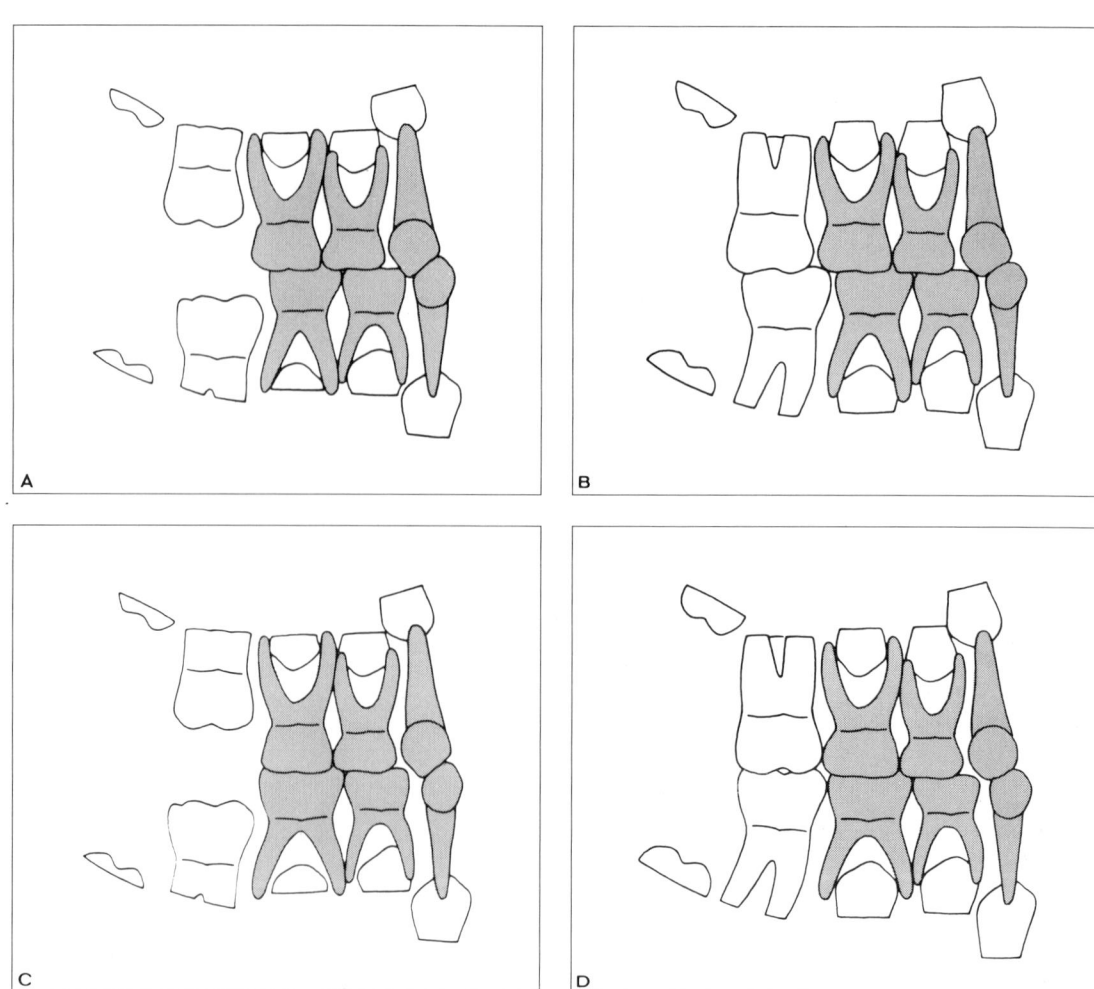

Figure 4-1

lost prematurely or the mesiodistal dimensions of their crowns are reduced by decay, other rules apply (Chapter 15).

The transition of the mandibular and maxillary incisors is explained in Figure 4-2. In this illustration, the teeth have been drawn in one plane. Such a representation has a disadvantage in that it is difficult to gain a good impression of the spatial relations. The inclination of the erupting teeth and the relation between the forming permanent teeth and their predecessors are difficult to grasp. The connection between the tooth dimensions and the size of the associated region in both jaws is not detectable, and differences in size and shape of the lower and upper jaw do not appear. For the indispensable three-dimensional insight in the transition of the mandibular and maxillary incisors, reference is made to the Atlas of van der Linden and Duterloo.[107]

The localization of the forming permanent incisors and canines within the jaws is determined in part by the size of the regions of the jaws in which these teeth are

Fig. 4-1 Influence of the mesiodistal crown dimensions of opposing second deciduous molars on the terminal plane of the deciduous dentition and on the position of the first permanent molars before and after emergence.

A *Situation at about 4 years of age with opposing second deciduous molars of approximately the same mesiodistal crown dimensions. Under normal conditions, the terminal plane will have a mesial step. The sagittal relation between the adjacent, not yet erupted first permanent molars corresponds. The mandibular one is slightly more ventrally positioned than the maxillary one.*
B *Upon emergence at about 6 years of age, the first permanent molars may attain maximal intercuspation immediately. The sagittal relation between the mandibular and maxillary first permanent molars, conforms to the situation normally present in the dentition of a young adult, when all permanent teeth have attained occlusion.*
C *Developmental stage corresponding to the one shown in A. The mesiodistal crown dimension of the mandibular second deciduous molar is a few millimeters larger than that of the maxillary one. The opposing second deciduous molars occlude normally and demonstrate the associated mesial shoulder at their mesial surfaces. However, because of the excess in mesiodistal crown width of the mandibular second deciduous molar, the terminal plane is flush. The sagittal relation of the not yet erupted first permanent molars conforms; they are oriented in an end-to-end position.*
D *After emergence, the first permanent molars do not attain maximal contact. However, a more or less correct transverse relation is established because the large mesiopalatal cusp of the maxillary first permanent molar becomes guided between the buccal and lingual cusps of the mandibular one by means of the cone-funnel mechanism (see Fig. 2-2). The maxillary first permanent molar becomes slightly more buccally placed than its antagonist. In mesiodistal direction, the two teeth are in an end-to-end relation.*
Not before the deciduous molars are replaced by the premolars can good sagittal relation and maximal contact and intercuspation of the first permanent molars be achieved. The mandibular first permanent molar is then able to migrate mesially over a larger distance than the maxillary one as the crowns of the opposing premolars have by and large the same mesiodistal crown dimensions. The difference of the deciduous molars in this respect provides the extra space needed for an improvement of the occlusion of the first permanent molars.

placed and in part by the dimensions of their crowns. The initial formation of the different teeth starts at varying height levels. The height of these levels is maintained during further formation until active tooth movement toward the occlusal plane begins. The variation in height levels of tooth formation is reflected in the ultimate length of the individual teeth. The canines are the longest teeth in the complete permanent dentition; they are formed at the greatest distance from the occlusal plane. Initially, the mandibular permanent canines are located closely to the cortical wall on the lower border of the mandible; the maxillary ones are adjacent to the piriform aperture. As such, the forming maxillary canines are at a larger distance from the occlusal plane than the central incisors, which are formed inferiorly to and in close proximity to the nasal floor. The maxillary lateral incisors are formed even more inferiorly and attain smaller ultimate tooth lengths than the central ones.
An adequate impression of the variation in height levels on which the formation of the

The First Transitional Period

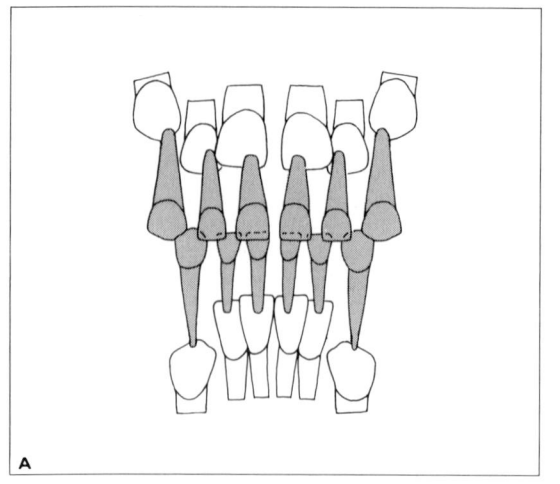
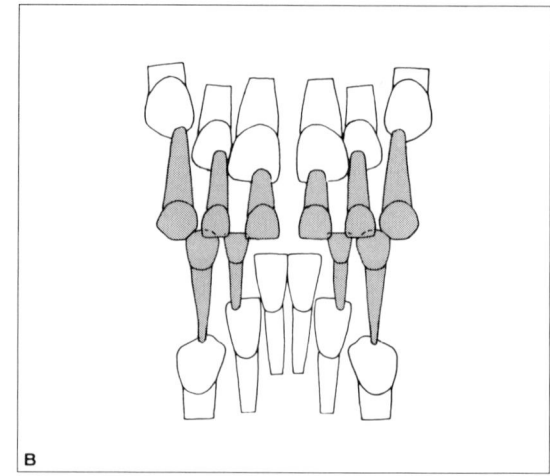
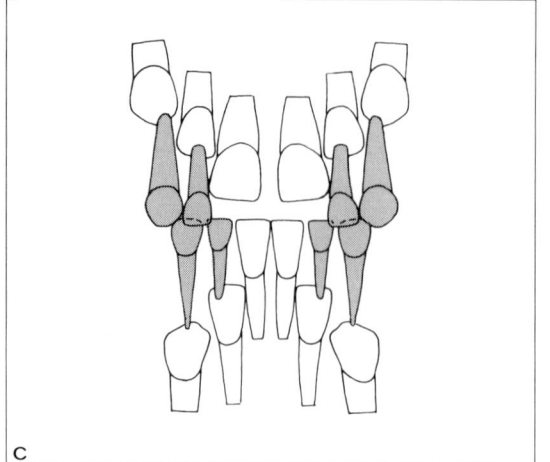
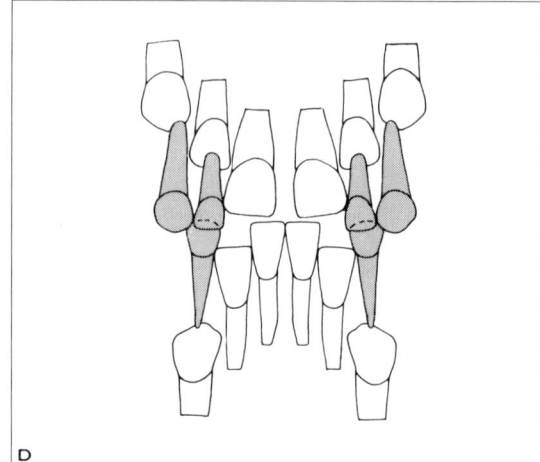
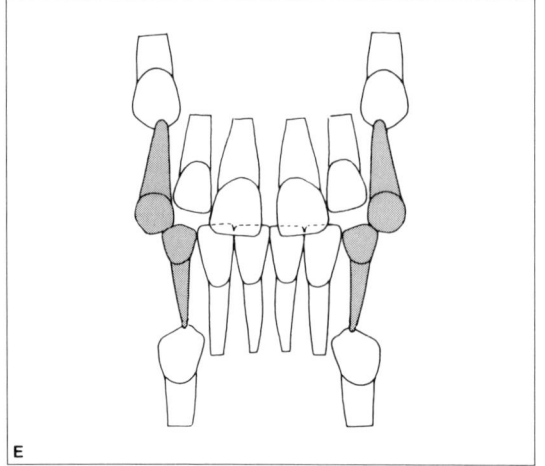
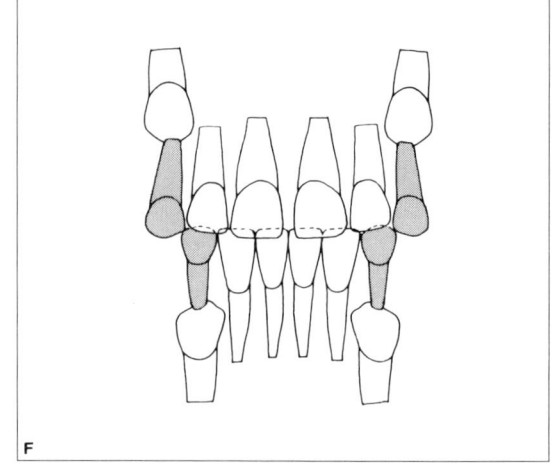

Figure 4-2

Fig. 4-2 Survey of the normal transition of the incisors by means of drawings representing the incisors and canines of both dentitions in one plane.

A Situation at approximately 5 years of age, prior to beginning of eruption of the permanent incisors. The differences in height of the permanent teeth have changed little since formation started. The incisal edges of the maxillary lateral permanent incisors are situated nearer the occlusal plane than those of the central ones. The distoincisal corners of the maxillary central permanent incisors are in contact with the mesial surfaces of the roots of the adjacent deciduous laterals. In the lower jaw, the incisal edges of the centrals are slightly nearer to the occlusal plane than those of the laterals. Here, the crowns of the permanent centrals are situated lingually to the roots of their predecessors and partly overlap the lingually located crowns of the permanent laterals. In both jaws, the amount of overlap of the central and lateral incisor crowns depends mainly on the relation between their mesiodistal crown dimensions on the one side and the space available within the jaws on the other side.[5] The localization of the crowns of the forming canines determines the lateral demarcations of the space available for the permanent incisors.[109]

B The mandibular central deciduous incisors shed first. Some time later, their successors emerge. In their eruption* movement, they pass the laterals. The contact between the distoincisal corners of the maxillary central permanent incisors and the mesial surfaces of the roots of the adjacent lateral deciduous incisors results in a distal displacement of the latter. The diastemata mesial to the maxillary deciduous canines reduce in width, and more space becomes available in the dental arch for the central permanent incisor crowns still to emerge. This increase in available space is needed as the crowns of the central permanent incisors have substantially larger mesiodistal crown dimensions than those of their predecessors.
The mandibular synchondrosis originally present at birth has disappeared; no remnants are left. The synostosis has been established and the previously morphologically distinguishable left and right mandibular sides form a solid bony unity. The left and right mandibular central permanent incisors can be positioned in close proximity before emergence, as is often the case.
Such a close proximity never exists in the maxilla, as the median suture persists until the development of the dentition is completed, as has been explained.
Because the mandibular central permanent incisors start to erupt some time before the lateral ones, the overlapping of the mandibular permanent incisor crowns is eliminated before the central ones have reached the level of the occlusal plane.

C The maxillary central deciduous incisors are lost and their successors have erupted further. The associated distal movement of the maxillary lateral deciduous incisors has continued, and the diastemata mesial to the deciduous canines now are closed. The descent of the maxillary central permanent incisors without a concomitant movement of the lateral ones leads to the elimination of the overlap of the crowns. In the mandible, the central permanent incisors have reached the level of the occlusal plane before the lateral ones begin to erupt. Occasionally, the eruption of the lateral begins earlier. In normal situations, adequate space is available in the mandibular dental arch and the crowns of the erupting permanent centrals do not contact the mesial surfaces of the adjacent deciduous laterals. However, when space is limited, a process comparable to that described above for the maxilla may take place. The crowns of the erupting centrals then will contact the mesial surfaces of the roots of the laterals and the latter will become displaced distally. The diastemata mesial to the deciduous canines reduce in width.

D The emerging maxillary central permanent incisors continue to move the deciduous lateral ones distally. This, in turn causes movement of the deciduous canines, resulting in an increase in intercanine distance. In the mandible, the erupting lateral permanent incisor crowns reach the deciduous canines, and their distoincisal corners make contact with the mesial surfaces of the latter. Subsequently, the mandibular intercanine distance increases. The two processes leading to an increase in intercanine distance in both jaws run approximately parallel in time. In accordance with this coincidence, observations have been made in longitudinal studies that the enlargement in intercanine width in the two dental arches occurs simultaneously.[7,8,63,64,72] Normally, maxillary central permanent incisors emerge with space between them (central diastema). In comparison with the mandibular central permanent incisors the lateral ones emerge more lingually than where their predecessors were located. Thus, the mandibular laterals emerge more lingually in the dental arch than do the centrals.

*See note on page 33.

E The maxillary lateral permanent incisors do not begin to erupt before the central ones have reached the level of the occlusal plane. Then they are able to erupt from their more lingual position (in comparison with the centrals) in a more labial direction toward the occlusal plane. If the crowns of the maxillary permanent laterals make contact with those of the centrals, the central diastema reduces in width.[21,22] However, this reduction also takes place when that contact is not established, as is more often the case.[5,45] Upon eruption of the maxillary laterals, more space becomes available in the region of the incisor roots. The apices of the centrals can move distally and their mesiodistal angulation changes accordingly. Their crowns will approach each other.

F The maxillary lateral permanent incisors reach the level of the occlusal plane last. Then the first transitional period is completed and the intertransitional period commences. Often diastemata are present in the maxillary anterior region, sometimes in the mandibular one. The roots of the maxillary lateral permanent incisors are in close proximity to the crowns of the permanent canines. This relation changes when the latter begin to erupt.

Functional influences exerted on the dentition by the tongue, the lips, and the buccal musculature play an important role in the transition of the incisors. These influences are not illustrated and discussed here. The same applies to the effect of abnormal habits (digit sucking) on the eruption and position of the anterior teeth. However, some of the aspects involved are treated in Figure 4-3 and more extensively in Chapter 16.

different teeth has started can be gained, with exception of the third molars, by looking at the height levels on which the incisal edges and cusp tips have been situated prior to the beginning of their active movements towards the occlusal plane (Fig. 4-2A). Further, it is assumed that a comparison of the lengths of completely formed permanent teeth can provide information in retrospect about the variation that existed in height levels of formation (see Fig. 8-5). In this, one has to keep in mind that not all permanent teeth are formed at the same time and that the duration of their formation varies. The maxillary central permanent incisor precedes the adjacent lateral in initiation of calcification, although the latter is located closer to the occlusal plane. The maxillary permanent canine is formed later than the lateral incisor; however, the former is situated considerably more superiorly.

The replacement of the deciduous teeth by the permanent ones takes place in two distinctly separated phases. In the *first transitional period* the incisors are exchanged. In the *second transitional period* the deciduous canines and molars are superseded by their successors. In between lies the *intertransitional period*, which lasts about 1.5 years.

A marked dissimilarity exists between the two transitional periods, caused mainly by differences in morphological conditions in the anterior and posterior regions. Some aspects of this dissimilarity will be elaborated here. The crowns of the permanent incisors are substantially larger than those of the corresponding deciduous teeth. Further, the permanent incisors are situated lingually to their predecessors. The forming parts are situated in the region where the roots of the fully erupted teeth will be located later. This region is smaller than the one formed later by the incisor crowns when they have reached the level of the occlusal plane. The segment formed by the crowns of the fully erupted permanent incisors and canines is larger than the one then formed by the apices of these teeth. This difference is more marked for the maxilla than for the mandible, in part because the permanent crowns of the maxillary permanent incisors and canines are larger than those of the mandibular ones, and partly because the space that contains the apices in the maxilla is located more dorsally than the one in the mandible.

The situation in the posterior region is different. The forming premolars are located between and below, or above the roots of their predecessors. Further, the premolars have a smaller mesiodistal crown dimension than their predecessors. Moreover, the area where the apices of the mandibular premolars will be located after complete eruption and attainment of occlusion is situated about perpendicularly below the area where the crowns will be placed. In the upper jaw a comparable but less favorable situation exists as the premolars will ultimately attain a slight buccal inclination. However, the difference in inclination between the premolar and incisors is still larger in the upper than in the lower jaw, as the maxillary incisors are considerably more labially inclined than their mandibular counterparts (see Fig. 7-2). The inclination of the permanent incisors in both jaws differs markedly from that of their predecessors, which, as explained, were about perpendicularly oriented to the occlusal plane. The space containing the apices of the deciduous incisors and canines at the complete deciduous dentition stage is only slightly smaller than that which will house the apices of their fully erupted successors later. As the permanent incisors are initially located lingually to the roots of their predecessors, the latter have to be in a more or less perpendicular position with their roots rather labially.

The transition of the incisors is a complex process. Many variations encountered will not be discussed here. For more information, refer to the literature[5,6,65,109]. The normal transition of the incisors is shown in Figure 4-2. The changes taking place in the sagittal plane through the mandibular and maxillary right central incisors and in the relation of these teeth to the lips are indicated in Figure 4-3, together with the changes in position of the mandibular and maxillary right first permanent molars and their mutual relation.

The loss of a deciduous tooth is caused by resorption of its root and, to a lesser extent, by reduction of bone that surrounds the deciduous root cervically. Both processes start rather early. At 4 years of age, parts of the roots of the mandibular and maxillary central deciduous incisors already have been resorbed and portions of the roots are no longer covered cervically by bone. When a deciduous tooth is shed, part of the alveolar process that surrounded the root disappears. During the eruption of the successors, the alveolar process that will surround its root is gradually built up again. An erupting permanent tooth partly creates its own alveolar process by means of osteogenic activity of its periodontal membrane and of the periosteum on the adjacent buccal and lingual surfaces.

The First Transitional Period

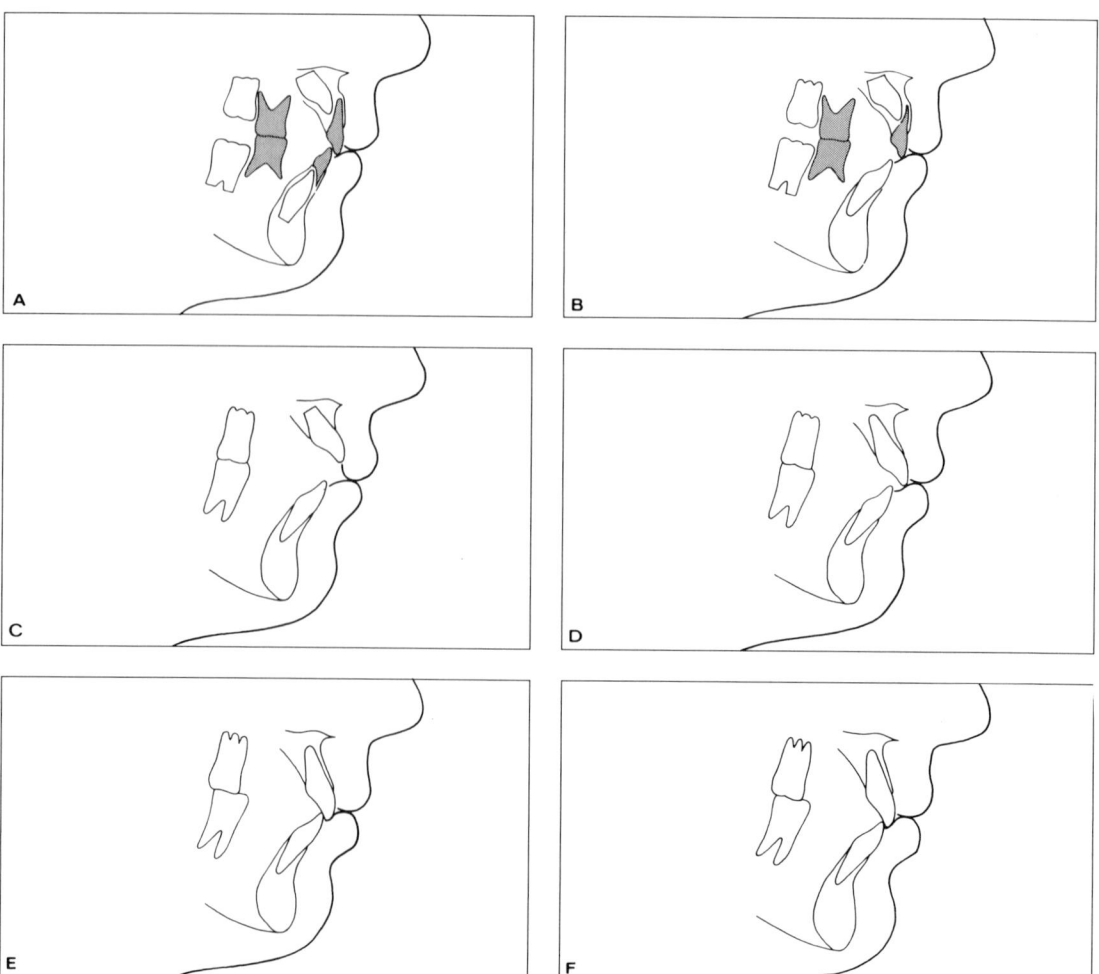

Fig. 4-3 Survey of the changes in the incisor and the molar region from the complete deciduous dentition stage to the adult situation. The drawings have been composed from cross sections through the right molars, the right central incisors and surrounding bony structures, and the profile.

A   In the complete deciduous dentition, the deciduous incisors are oriented approximately perpendicularly to the occlusal plane. The permanent incisors are located lingually to the roots of their predecessors and are labially inclined. The resorption of the roots of the deciduous teeth is associated with the eruption of their successors.

B   The mandibular first permanent molar is the first permanent tooth to emerge, followed by the mandibular central incisor. After emergence, the mandibular central permanent incisor continues its eruption in the same direction as before, which is in accordance with its original localization within the jaw. The maxillary central permanent incisor, which also maintains its original inclination within the jaw during its pre-emergence eruption process,[95] has erupted further and concomitantly the resorption of the root of its predecessor has proceeded. The lower lip touches the incisal edge of the maxillary deciduous incisors and covers the labial surface slightly.

C   The maxillary first permanent molar has emerged and attained contact with its antagonist. The intercuspation is not maximal in this case as the distal surfaces of the second deciduous molars *(not drawn) have a flush terminal plane. The first permanent molars occlude sagittally in an end-to-end relation. The first permanent molars will not establish solid intercuspation before the transition of the posterior teeth is completed (E). The mandibular central incisor erupts further and the maxillary one emerges several weeks to a few months after the shedding of its predecessor. Part of the alveolar bone surrounding the incisor will be reconstructed during the eruption process. The bone around the remnants of the deciduous root has disappeared before shedding.*

D *In its eruption after emergence, the position of the mandibular incisors is influenced by the tongue and lower lip. The upper lip makes contact with the maxillary incisors shortly after their emergence. The inclination of the maxillary incisors is influenced by the upper lip, resulting in a reduction of its labial inclination.*

E *The mandibular and maxillary permanent incisors continue to erupt until mutual support is established by occlusal contact. The maxillary right central incisor is not only supported vertically by the two contacting mandibular right incisors, but also by the lower lip. The latter touches the incisal edge of the maxillary central incisors and covers its labial surface vertically over a distance of 1 to 3 mm. Not only the upper lip but also the lower lip exerts a force in the lingual direction on the maxillary central incisors. In addition, the lower lip makes contact with the mandibular incisors.*

F *After years, the maxillary and mandibular incisors have attained a steeper inclination in the adult situation. This change is associated with the continuation of jaw growth after the permanent teeth have established occlusion. The pressure exerted by the peri-oral musculature on the incisors also plays a role in the realization of this change in inclination.*

As a rule, in both jaws several weeks to a few months will pass before the shedding of a deciduous incisor is followed by the emergence of its successor. This interval is related in part to the reconstruction of the alveolar process indicated above and partly to the healing of the gingival defect that is present after a tooth has been lost. In addition, there is usually some delay due to the fact that the successor has to perforate the overlying gingival tissue.

One month or more may pass between the emergence of a corresponding left and right incisor in one jaw. Asymmetry in this respect is encountered less in the mandible than in the maxilla. A permanent tooth starts its eruption movement after one quarter of its ultimate root length has been attained. The predecessor becomes more rapidly resorbed. Permanent teeth perforate the gingival tissue and appear in the oral cavity when the roots are formed to three-fourths of their length.[67,76]

A small opening in the bony alveolar process is present on the lingual side of each deciduous incisor in the lower and upper jaws. This opening forms the oral aspect of the gubernacular canal, which runs to the crypt of the successor. Originally the gubernacular canal contains the gubernacular cord, which initially consists of epithelium of the dental lamina. The epithelium dissolves and a connective tissue strand remains, which subsequently disintegrates further.[11] The opening of the gubernacular canal on the oral side increases in size with the approach of the associated permanent tooth. The gubernacular canal probably plays a role in the guidance of the direction of eruption of the incisors through the bone and in the determination of the spot of emergence.[107] Permanent incisors seem to perforate the bone surface where the oral opening of the gubernacular canal originally had been located lingually to the place where their predecessors had been situated.

The First Transitional Period

A permanent tooth tends to erupt in a direction which conforms to its initial position within the jaw. Upon emergence, a permanent tooth migrates to its future location in the dental arch. A maxillary lateral permanent incisor erupts in a more labial direction than the central one has done. After the lateral incisor has emerged and further erupted, its labial inclination becomes gradually reduced. A mandibular lateral permanent incisor emerges lingually in the dental arch. Subsequently it moves labially under the influence of pressures exerted by the tongue and finally becomes positioned harmoniously within the dental arch. Generally, the process of eruption following emergence is influenced by environmental factors. The most important factors in this respect are the local space conditions in the dental arches and the position and functional activity of the tongue and of the lips and buccal musculature.

The complete process of the transition of the mandibular and maxillary incisors takes more than three years starting with the first changes taking place in the deciduous dental arch (Figs. 4-2A and B) through the full eruption of all permanent incisors (Figs. 4-2E and F). The distal movement of the maxillary lateral deciduous incisors associated with the transition starts more than one year prior to the emergence of the permanent central incisors. As such, this movement precedes the loss of the mandibular central deciduous incisors and the subsequent emergence of their successors. In each jaw, about 12 months pass between the emergence of the central permanent incisors and the laterals. Thus, the emergence of the maxillary central permanent incisors coincides approximately with that of the mandibular lateral ones. About 8 months pass between the emergence of an incisor in the oral cavity and the attainment of full eruption.[39] For more details, information on average emergence times, and more numerical data, refer to Chapter 17.

Chapter 5

The Dentition in the Intertransitional Period

In the intertransitional period the mandibular and maxillary dental arches consist of sets of deciduous and permanent teeth. Between the four permanent incisors and the left and right first permanent molars, the deciduous canines and first and second deciduous molars are located on each side of the dental arch. The maxillary incisors are labially inclined. A central diastema is present. Frequently no contact exists either between the central and lateral incisors. Likewise, a diastema is often present in the maxillary dental arch mesially to the deciduous canine. In the mandible the incisors are less labially inclined than in the maxilla. A diastema seldom exists between the mandibular central incisors. All incisor crowns are usually in contact with each other and the laterals touch the deciduous canine crowns.

The arrangement of incisors in the intertransitional period deviates from the normal situation in the adult dentition when all incisors are well aligned and in contact with each other. However, the marked, unharmonious-appearing situation characteristic of the preceding first transitional period has disappeared for the greater part. Asymmetry in emergence and associated differences in height levels and lengths of clinical crowns of corresponding left and right teeth have been made up. Under the influence of the tongue, the mandibular lateral incisors have attained the proper sites within the dental arch and their initially lingual location has been eliminated. Small rotations resulting from rotated positions of the tooth buds—quite often encountered in the mandible—are corrected by pressures exerted by the tongue and lips if the spatial conditions in the dental arch permit these improvements to be achieved. The incisal contacts between the maxillary and mandibular incisors also may work in favor of this improvement.

The deciduous teeth still present are normally quite worn down at this developmental stage. The initially present sharp cusp tips of the deciduous canines and molars have disappeared by attrition and the occlusal morphology approaches that of a plane. Through the absence of a distinct intercuspation, the anteroposterior relation between the two jaws is not fixed by the occlusion anymore. The ventral development of the mandible, slightly exceeding that of the maxilla, encounters little or no interferences from the occlusal contacts, so the mandibular teeth attain a slightly more mesial position in relation to the maxillary ones.

Not only the occlusal, but also the approximal surfaces wear off in normal use through rubbing the adjacent surfaces during function. The initially pointed

The Intertransitional Period

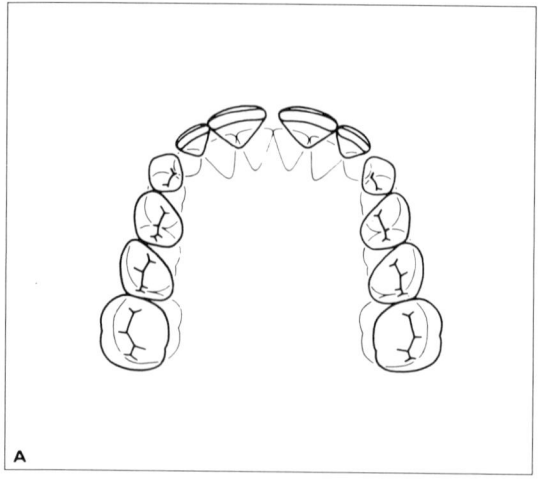
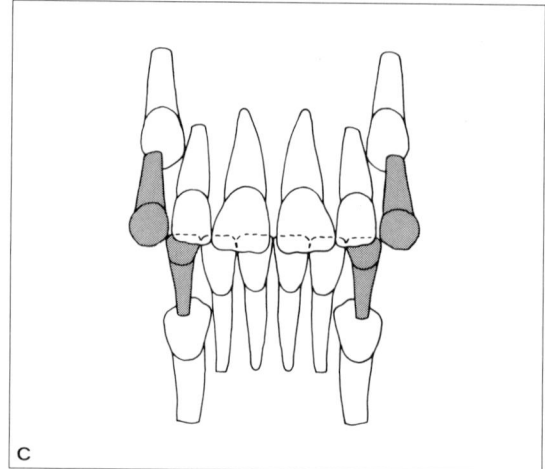
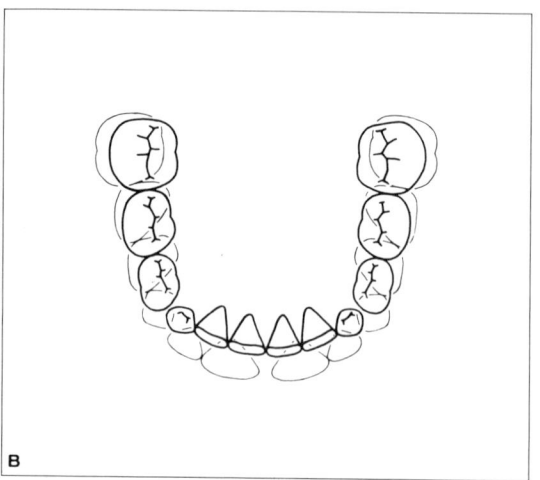
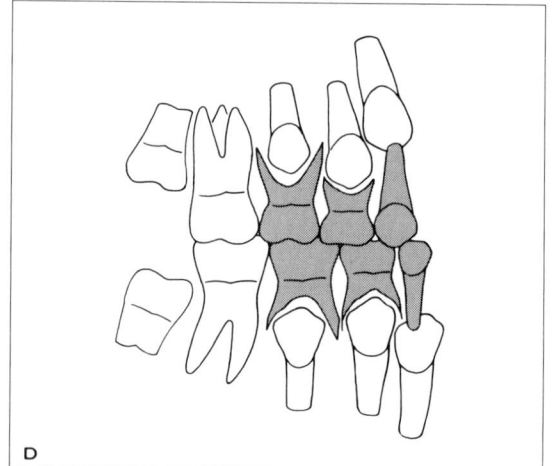

Fig. 5-1 Survey of the normal situation of the dentition in the intertransitional period.

The occlusal patterns are only drawn in the maxillary (A) or only in the mandibular (B) teeth to facilitate the identification of the different teeth and to improve the proper evaluation of their positions. In studying this illustration and comparable ones to follow, it must be realized that the original occlusal morphology of the deciduous molars has disappeared for the greater part by the time the intertransitional period is reached. The cusps are worn and the occlusal morphology of the deciduous molars approaches that of a plane. Intercuspation has disappeared accordingly. At the mesial and distal surfaces, attrition also has occurred. The contact points drawn in these and comparable illustrations are in reality contact planes.

A   Together, the maxillary teeth form a harmonious dental arch. Practically always a diastema is present between the central incisors. Sometimes the adjacent central and lateral incisors are in contact. Between the latter and the deciduous canines, a diastema often exists. The first permanent molar is located distally to the second deciduous molar. Initially, space exists between these teeth after emergence of the former. After some time, contact usually is attained between the second deciduous molar and the first permanent molar. The maxillary teeth occlude slightly buccally with the mandibular ones. The overjet of the incisors is larger than it was in the

The Intertransitional Period

deciduous dentition and also larger than it will be when the permanent dentition is completed and the growth of the jaws has terminated (compare Fig. 4-3).

B The mandibular dental arch is also harmoniously shaped. Usually, only a few diastemata are present and these are concentrated mainly between the deciduous canines and the first deciduous molars, the embrasures opposing the maxillary deciduous canines.

Most often, the first permanent molars do not occlude well at this developmental stage. No solid contact and intercuspation have yet developed in sagittal direction. The mesiodistal crown dimensions of the second deciduous molars play an essential role in this respect as has been explained in Chapter 4 and particularly in Figure 4-1.

C The four maxillary incisors contact the four mandibular incisors and canines in occlusion. The incisal edges of the four mandibular incisors are at the same height. In the maxillary dental arch the incisal edges of the centrals are slightly inferior to those of the laterals.

The crowns of the not yet emerged permanent canines limit the space available for the roots of the mandibular and maxillary incisors. The roots of the laterals converge apically. This convergence is more distinct in the upper than in the lower jaw.

D Through the attrition of the occlusal surfaces, the intercuspation of the deciduous molars is largely lost. The sagittal relation between the two dental arches is only slightly fixed by the occlusal contact of the deciduous molars or not at all. During the intertransitional period, a sagittal fixation between the two dental arches, based on intercuspation, is usually lacking. Such a fixation was provided earlier by the intercuspation of the not yet abraded deciduous molars and will be provided later by the strong intercuspation of the premolars and permanent canines that fit together in the style of gear wheels. The attrition of the deciduous molars allows a slight change in sagittal direction between the two dental arches, if the ventral development of the lower jaw exceeds that of the upper. This change in sagittal relation, although slight, usually takes place in the complete deciduous dentition, in the first transitional stage as well as in the intertransitional period.

Resorption of the roots of the deciduous molars and of the interlying bone provides the space for the eruption of the premolars. The patterns of resorption conform to the morphology of the premolar crowns. The resorbing deciduous molar roots and the adjacent bone form, as it were, enlarged impressions (negatives) of the premolar crowns.

The space available for the premolars and permanent canines is less in the maxilla than in the mandible. This dissimilarity is associated with the larger mesiodistal crown dimensions of the mandibular deciduous molar crowns in comparison with those of the maxillary ones and with the difference in size and morphology of the bony structures in which the premolars and permanent canines are localized in both jaws.

At this stage, the second permanent molars are located within the jaws dorsally to the not yet solid occluding first permanent molars. The occlusal surface of the maxillary second permanent molar is oriented in a distal and buccal direction; that of the mandibular in a mesial and lingual direction. The prior-to-emergence localization of the second permanent molars reflects the restricted spatial conditions within the jaws.

approximal contacts become flat and the mesiodistal crown dimensions reduce in size. These changes caused by attrition are limited in modern Western societies. However, in a life-style that requires greater activity and a more vigorous functioning of the dentition, and one that involves exposure to materials with a rather large abrading effect, as grains of sand, the attrition will be considerably larger. It has been assumed that deciduous molars need the excess in mesiodistal crown dimensions over their successors to be able to maintain the space needed for the premolars even after considerable approximal attrition.[43]

The mesiodistal angulation of the mandibular and maxillary permanent incisors is determined partly by the position of the permanent canine crowns that have not yet emerged. The latter are in close proximity to the roots of the lateral incisors, which usually converge apically. Not until the permanent canines have emerged and erupted further does space become available within the jaws for the distal movement of the apices of the lateral incisors. The initially apical convergence of the roots of the lateral incisors and the changes in angulation following the emergence of the permanent canines is more explicit in the maxilla than in the mandible.

Root formation of already emerged incisors and molars continues during the intertransitional period. This also applies to teeth that have not yet emerged. The roots of the permanent canines, premolars, and second permanent molars gradually increase in length. The space needed for that purpose is provided by the concomitantly occurring increase in height of the alveolar processes in both jaws.

The roots of the deciduous molars resorb simultaneously with the movement of the premolars in the occlusal direction. Part of the bone cervically surrounding the roots of the deciduous molars gradually disappears also. A comparable process takes place around the roots of the deciduous canines. The resorption pattern of the deciduous canines conforms more to that of the deciduous incisors, although the former usually resorb more horizontally than from the lingual side because the permanent canines are placed more apically to their predecessors than is the case for the incisors.

The intertransitional period presents itself in a growing child as a rather stable phase with little changes in the dentition. At least this impression is gained when only the intra-oral picture is considered. However, within the jaws, the processes described above—resorption of the deciduous roots and reduction in the cervically surrounding bone—take place. The second transitional period is prepared by these processes. This also holds true for the continuing formation of the permanent teeth still to emerge. Their roots increase in length and the crown of the third molars, if present, starts to calcify. This calcification of a third molar happens at approximately the same time as the furcation of the adjacent second permanent molar is formed. In accordance with the overall precedence of lower jaw dentition development over the upper one, mandibular third molars start to calcify before their maxillary counterparts. The situation of the dentition in the intertransitional period is illustrated in Figure 5-1; a sagittal cross section is shown in Figure 4-3E. To gain a better perspective of the three-dimensional aspects in the localization of the teeth within the jaws and their mutual relations, refer to the Atlas of van der Linden and Duterloo.[107]

Chapter 6

The Transition of the Posterior Teeth and the Emergence of the Second Permanent Molars—The Second Transitional Period

At approximately 10 years of age the first deciduous tooth in the posterior regions—usually a mandibular canine—sheds. This happens more than 1.5 years after the maxillary lateral incisor has emerged as the last of the permanent incisors and about one year after it has reached the level of the occlusal plane. In contrast to the situation for the incisors, a marked variation exists in the shedding sequence of the posterior teeth and the emergence of their successors. A deviating sequence of emergence normally does not occur in both anterior regions, as the localization of the permanent incisors prior to the beginning of eruption and the spatial conditions within the jaws impede this. A comparable impediment does not exist for the mandibular and maxillary posterior regions as the permanent teeth are further apart prior to emergence and no crowding exists within the jaws. An exception in this respect is the relation between the first premolar and permanent canine in the maxilla. During formation, these teeth are in close proximity to each other and overlap vertically. The already calcified distal corner of the permanent canine is directly adjacent to the forming mesial cervical region of the first premolar. Accordingly, the maxillary first premolar shows a concavity on the mesial surface at the cementoenamel junction (*fossa canina*). A comparable mesial concavity is absent, or present only in reduced form, at the maxillary second premolar whose crown morphology strongly resembles that of the maxillary first premolar. Conforming to the mutual relation between the maxillary permanent canine and first premolar described above, the premolar erupts first. As a rule, only when the spatial conditions are so ample that the situation is comparable to the one in the mandible can the maxillary permanent canine emerge prior to the first premolar. Under these conditions the maxillary first premolar does not act as an obstacle for the descent of the permanent canine.

The most frequently occurring sequence of emergence of the posterior permanent teeth with predecessors in the mandible is (1) canine, (2) first premolar, and (3) second premolar. In the maxilla it is (1) first premolar, (2) second premolar, and (3) canine.[54] These sequences are applied in the design of Figure 6-1, which

The Second Transitional Period

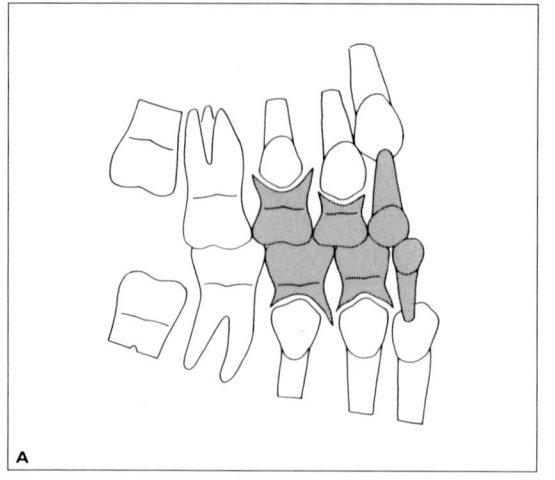
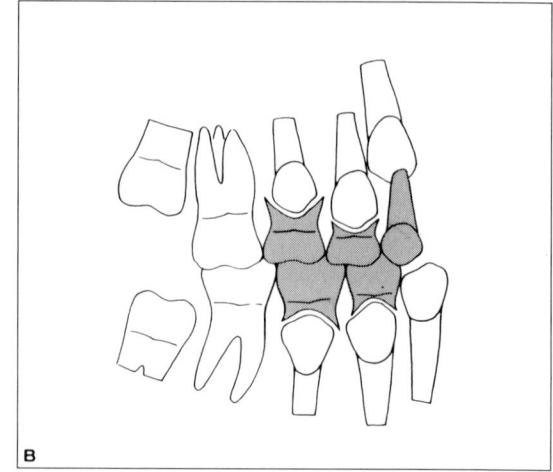
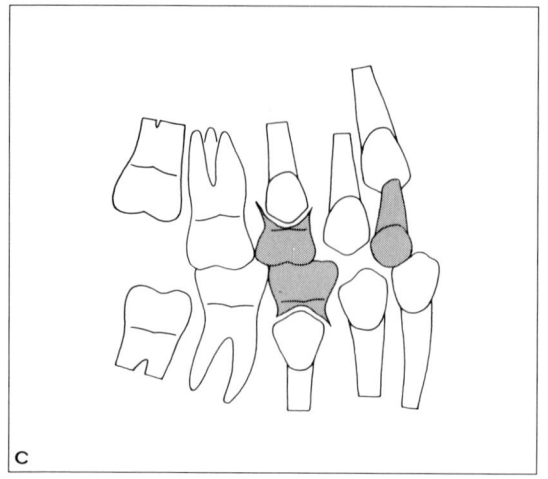
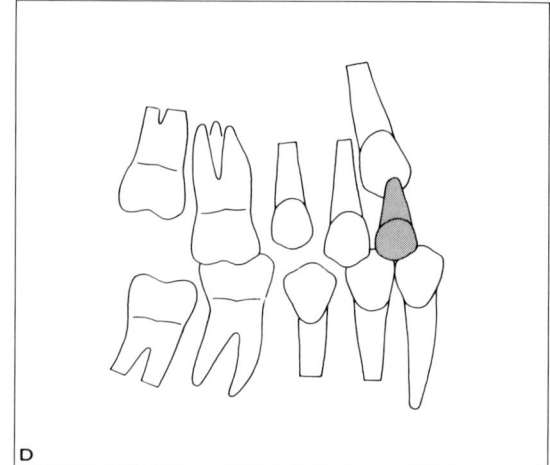
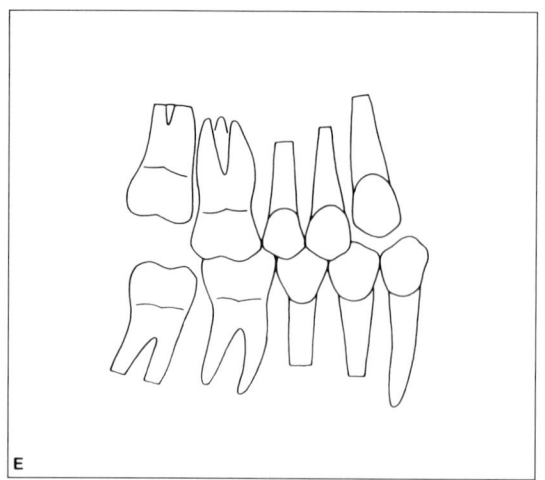
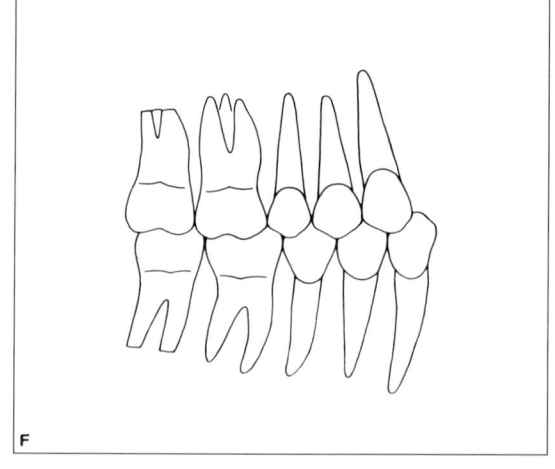

Figure 6-1

Fig. 6-1 Survey of the transition of the posterior teeth and the eruption of the second permanent molars.

A The premolar crowns are located between the roots of their predecessors, which resorb in concert with the continuing eruption of the premolars. In the maxilla, the first premolar is nearest to the occlusal plane and the permanent canine is farthest away. The distal corner of the permanent canine is located in close proximity to the concavity at the mesial cementoenamel junction of the adjacent first premolar (fossa canina). A comparable concavity has not developed on the second premolars or has developed only slightly. In vertical direction, the second premolar is located between the first premolar and the permanent canine. Also in the lower jaw, the permanent canine is initially farther from the occlusal plane than the first premolar (see Fig. 4-1). However, both teeth are situated somewhat apart, unlike the situation in the upper jaw. Their mesiodistal angulation is about perpendicular to the occlusal plane, as is the case for the mandibular second premolar. The corresponding maxillary teeth are angulated slightly mesially.

In this drawing, the mandibular second deciduous molar has only a slightly larger mesiodistal crown dimension than its antagonist. Accordingly, the terminal plane shows a distinct mesial step. Hence, the first permanent molars intercuspate in maximal contact, and a solid sagittal occlusion exists.

The second permanent molars are distobuccally oriented in the maxilla and mesiolingually in the mandible, in conformity with the local spatial conditions in both jaws and the original location of the forming parts of these teeth.

In both jaws, the apices of the first permanent molars and the forming parts of the other permanent teeth are oriented in approximately one plane. Only the forming parts of the permanent canines, particularly in the maxilla, are located farther from the occlusal plane in accordance with the longer roots ultimately to be attained.

B Shortly after the mandibular deciduous canine is shed, its successor emerges as the first deciduous posterior tooth. In its eruption movement, the latter has passed the adjacent first premolar. Sufficient space is available in the dental arch for the emerging mandibular permanent canine to attain a good position. The extra space needed for the relatively large crown is partially provided by the diastema that was present distally to the deciduous canine. In the maxilla, the first premolar is further erupted than both adjacent permanent teeth. The first premolar has descended, lost contact with the permanent canine crown and more closely approached the crown of its predecessor.

C The first premolars in both jaws emerge shortly after the mandibular permanent canine did. They can attain a harmonious position in the dental arch because adequate space is available. Both second premolars and the maxillary permanent canine have continued their eruption and the roots of their predecessors have resorbed concomitantly.

D The roots of the second deciduous molars are almost completely resorbed by the time of shedding. The crown persists for some time as a hat on top of the already emerged successor. The second premolar continues to erupt further in the space excessively available in the dental arch. In cases with a good sagittal relation between the first permanent molars, as illustrated here, the intercuspation of these teeth will be maintained. However, in cases with a flush terminal plane due to an excess in mesiodistal crown dimension of the mandibular second deciduous molar in comparison with its antagonist, the associated end-to-end relation of the first permanent molars will change to a solid intercuspation by a more mesial migration of the mandibular first permanent molar than of the maxillary one after loss of the second deciduous molars.

E The maxillary deciduous canine is the last deciduous tooth to be lost. As in the mandible, the successor emerges shortly thereafter. The permanent canine can attain a good position in the dental arch. The extra space needed for its large crown is provided in part by the diastema that was originally present mesially to the deciduous canine and in part by reduction of the central diastema and those between the central and lateral incisors, if present. After the first contact has been reached, the further eruption of the premolars will be guided by their occlusal morphology. Usually the premolars become reciprocally displaced in mesiodistal and buccolingual directions during the process of attaining the correct intercuspation. Depending on a variety of factors, the excess of available space in the dental arches will be filled more from the distal or more from the mesial direction.

The Second Transitional Period

F The maxillary permanent canine has arrived at the proper place in the dental arch. The mandibular second permanent molar and subsequently the maxillary one have emerged. At emergence, the mandibular second permanent molar is mesiolingually oriented, the maxillary one distobuccally. By means of the cone-funnel mechanism (see Fig. 2-2), these teeth become more upright and gradually attain good intercuspation. In many cases the transition of the posterior teeth has not yet been completed when the second permanent molars emerge (Fig. 6-2).

The complete process of the transition of the posterior teeth lasts years. The sequence of replacement can vary considerably. All theoretically possible variations in eruption sequence actually do occur in the mandible. The same applies to the maxilla, with the restriction that seldom will the permanent canine emerge prior to the first premolar. Only when excess space is available in the areas of the jaw that contains the canine and the first premolar can the canine generally emerge before the first premolar.

The emergence of the second permanent molar can take place during or after completion of the transition of the posterior teeth. The mandibular second permanent molar usually erupts prior to the maxillary one, with an interval of a few months to half a year.

---

demonstrates the transition in the posterior regions and the emergence of the second permanent molars. The two teeth listed above as the first two to appear in each jaw may become visible in the mouth simultaneously or shortly after each other. In the mandible all types of variations may occur in the sequence of emergence of the permanent canine and the premolars. The same holds true for the maxilla with the restriction, indicated above, that as a rule the first premolar precedes the permanent canine in emergence. For frequences in occurrence of the different emergence sequences[46,73,87,98] as well as for average emergence times[44,106] and other relevant numerical information, refer to Chapter 17.

In the majority of cases the second permanent molar emerges after all deciduous teeth have been lost and replaced. However, in many cases the second permanent molar appears in the mouth while mesially the neighboring second deciduous molar is still present (Fig. 6-2).

In each jaw the times of transition of corresponding left and right teeth can vary considerably. Also, the sequence of emergence in the two sides of the jaw can be different. Moreover, the transition in the lower jaw usually runs ahead of that in the upper.

The effect of the difference in mesiodistal crown dimensions between opposing second deciduous molars on the occlusion of the first permanent molars prior to the transition in the posterior region is explained in Chapter 4. The combined sequences of transition of the posterior teeth in the mandible and the maxilla determine when a flush terminal plane will dissolve. This change generally does not occur before the mandibular second deciduous molar is shed and subsequently the occlusion of the permanent first molars can improve. In cases with a terminal plane with a distinct mesial step, a solid intercuspation of the permanent first molars usually is present prior to the transition of the posterior teeth. Under these conditions, a mesial migration of the mandibular first permanent molar in relation to the maxillary one is not needed and either will not occur or only slightly.

The mesiodistal crown dimensions of the premolars are smaller than those of their predecessors. This holds true particularly for the mandibular second premolar; somewhat less for the maxillary second premolar, and only slightly for the mandibular and maxillary first premolars. The reverse situation is present for the canines. The crown of the maxillary permanent canine is considerably broader than that of its predecessor. In the mandible the difference is less marked. In both dental arches, the extra space needed for the broader permanent canine crowns is usually present as diastemata prior to the loss of their predecessors. In addition, part of the extra space remaining after the replacement of the deciduous molars by the premolars can be used to improve the position of the canine if needed. Upon emergence of the canines the excess in space is larger in the mandible than in the maxilla. The conditions for a good alignment are therefore more favorable for the mandibular than for the maxillary canine.

Prior to transition, the permanent canine and premolars approach the crowns of their predecessors whose roots resorb concomitantly. Also, the reduction of the alveolar bone continues at the cervical border of the deciduous teeth that are going to be lost. The roots of the deciduous molars resorb almost completely. An erupting premolar moves up to the crown of its predecessor and finally enters it. The crown of a deciduous molar can appear as a hat on the premolar crown. Often the buccal surface of a premolar crown is visible prior to the loss of the covering deciduous molar crown. After loss of the latter, the former becomes exposed. No time interval elapses between the shedding of a deciduous molar and the emergence of the succeeding premolar, as is found in the transition of incisors. On the contrary, generally a premolar does not emerge after but prior to the loss of its predecessor. Another and probably associated difference with the situation at the incisors is that the gubernacular canal of the premolars does not end on the oral surface of the bony alveolar processes lingually to the predecessor, but lingually in its alveolus. In this respect the situation at the canines is comparable to the one at the incisors. At the canines the gubernacular canal ends lingually to the deciduous canine crown on the oral surface of the alveolar bone. Prior to the start of eruption, and thereafter, the cusp tip of the permanent canine in both jaws is positioned lingually to the root of its predecessor. On the other side, the buccal surface of the permanent canine crown is more buccally positioned than that of the corresponding deciduous canine crown and root. As such, the permanent canine crowns are distinctly manifest and palpable in both jaws prior to emergence. This phenomenon is related to the large buccal bulging of the permanent canine crown (particularly in the maxilla), and the inclination of this tooth within the jaw with the forming part of the root positioned only slightly lingually to the crown (particularly in the mandible).

The prior-to-emergence position of the premolars and permanent canines in the jaw already has been treated in Chapters 4 and 5. The more these teeth near the occlusal plane, the more they affect the oral morphology of the covering bony structures. Not only permanent canines, but also premolars, particularly the mandibular ones, become palpable.

In the same dental arch, the times of emergence of the first and second permanent molars are correlated more closely with those of the deciduous teeth than with those of the permanent ones that have predecessors (see Chapter 17). The deciduous

The Second Transitional Period

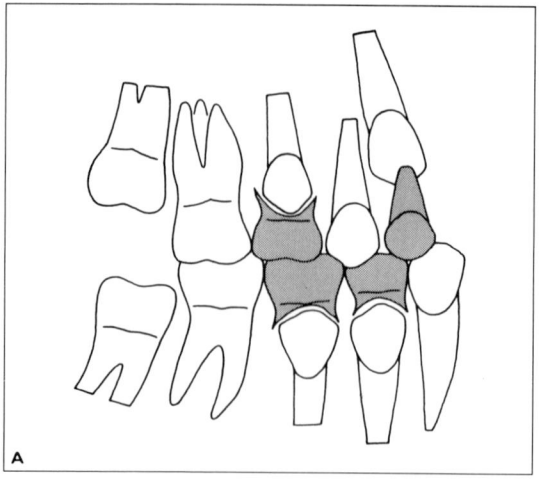
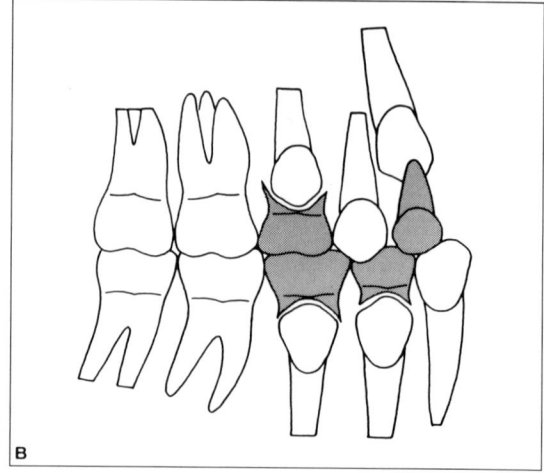
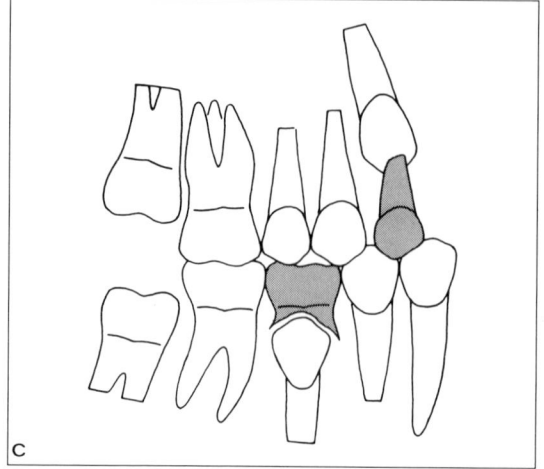
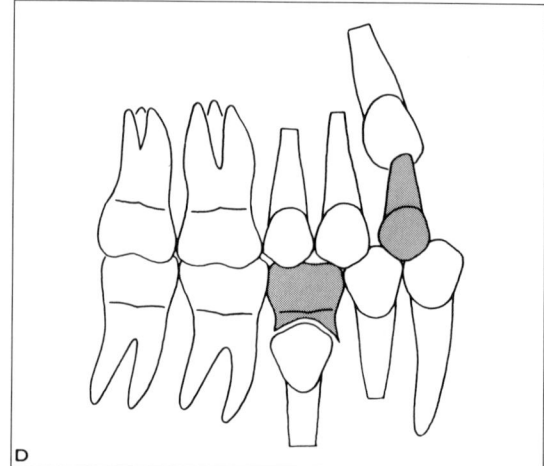

Figure 6-2

Fig. 6-2 Survey of some variations in the transition sequence of the posterior teeth and the emergence of the second permanent molars and in the shape of the terminal plane.

A   In the transition process, the mandibular permanent canine and the maxillary first premolar have emerged first and at about the same time. The second permanent molars have not yet emerged. The terminal plane shows a mesial step. The first permanent molars occlude adequately with a good intercuspation.

B   The emergence of the second permanent molars has taken place during or shortly after the transition of the mandibular canines and the replacement of the maxillary first deciduous molar by its successor. The mesial step of the terminal plane is limited in size. The first permanent molars occlude accordingly.

C   The mandibular permanent canine and first premolar have emerged simultaneously. The same applies to the two maxillary premolars. The second permanent molars have not yet emerged. The occlusion of the first permanent molars cannot improve until the mandibular second deciduous molar, with its extra large mesiodistal crown dimension, is lost.

D   The second permanent molars have emerged prior to the completion of the transition of the posterior teeth. Only the maxillary deciduous canine and the mandibular second deciduous molar remain to be replaced. The mesial surface of the mandibular first permanent molar is located slightly mesially to that of its antagonist. After the loss of the mandibular second deciduous molar, the first and second permanent molars can improve their occlusal relations.

---

teeth form a kind of unity with the permanent molars in this respect as also holds true for their morphogenesis, although in general, an early emergence of deciduous teeth is associated with an early transition and the reverse. However, the correlation between the emergence of the deciduous teeth and that of their successors is smaller than the correlation indicated above between the emergence of the first and second permanent molars and that of the deciduous teeth.[69] This difference in correlations is expressed in the variation in sequence of emergence of the second permanent molars and that of second premolars. Another factor that plays a role in this respect is the space available for emergence of the second permanent molar. A relatively late emergence of that tooth can be caused by lack of available space. Shortly before emergence, the second permanent molars are not oriented about perpendicularly to the occlusal plane as is the case for the first ones. The preceding dorsal enlargement of the tooth-bearing structures in both jaws has provided ample space for harmonious emergence of the first permanent molars. With decreasing jaw growth the space that becomes available for the second permanent molars prior to and upon emergence is more limited. Before emergence, the mandibular second permanent molar is oriented in a mesial and lingual direction, conforming to its initial orientation during formation. The area of the mandible where first the crown of the second permanent molar and afterwards its root are formed is situated relatively more to the buccal and dorsal side than the position that the crowns will occupy after occlusion has been attained. In the maxilla, the situation is reversed. The forming crown of the second permanent molar, and later its forming roots, are located rather palatally in close proximity to the roots of the first permanent molar. The occlusal surface is oriented in buccal and distal directions. After emergence, the opposing second permanent molars are guided into occlusion by the cone-funnel mechanism

(Fig. 2-2). Not until contact is attained do the teeth start to upright and gradually establish a good buccolingual inclination.

The situation prior to and after emergence of the maxillary second permanent molars, and later on also of the third molars, resembles the corresponding situation of the maxillary incisors in a certain way. Prior to emergence, the large crowns are accommodated in an area that afterwards only has to house the relatively narrower roots. After all pertaining teeth have emerged and fully erupted, the roots can become distributed in the available area. The mesiodistal angulation of the teeth changes accordingly. In the anterior region, the size of the area containing the incisor roots increases only slightly after the first permanent tooth has emerged. In the molar region, the dorsal extension continues and does not arrest until shortly before the termination of facial growth. The formation of the permanent molars proceeds accordingly, as has been explained before. Moreover, the interval in emergence times between subsequently emerging adjacent permanent molars is six years, not one year, as is the case for adjacent permanent incisors on one side of the jaw.

The transition of the posterior teeth and the eruption of the second permanent molars are complex and involve many three-dimensional features. For more details and a better insight, refer to the literature[4,103,105,109,110,112,113,114] and to the van der Linden and Duterloo Atlas.[107]

Chapter 7

The Permanent Dentition

The situation of the permanent dentition is discussed here only within the confines of the description of the final stage of the development of the dentition. Emphasis is placed in this respect on those facets of the permanent dentition that are thought to be able to clarify the preceding development. For information regarding the occlusion of the individual teeth, their function, and the physiology of the masticatory system, refer to appropriate textbooks.*
The position of the individual teeth in the permanent dentition, the relation between the dental arches, the occlusion and, in part, the spatial orientation are indicated in Figure 7-1.
At approximately 13 years of age all permanent teeth—except the eventually forming third molars—are fully erupted. Subsequently, their roots become more or less equally distributed over the available space within the jaws. This displacement of roots is gradual in nature, takes years to accomplish, and is mainly limited to the maxilla and the mandibular incisor region. The apices of the lateral incisors in the maxilla become distally displaced. Also in the maxillary posterior region, the spaces between the roots become more or less equally distributed over the available area. This process cannot be completed before the third molars have erupted fully. In case of missing third molars, the process may start earlier and be completed at a younger age. The apices of the maxillary second molar and also the first one can move distally, resulting in a change in orientation of these teeth. This change in orientation appears clinically by the development of mesial angulation of the maxillary first and second permanent molars. The distal marginal ridge of the maxillary first molar becomes more inferiorly positioned than the adjacent mesial marginal ridge of the second molar. The other teeth in the maxilla—with the exception of the second premolar— also demonstrate a mesial angulation. In the mandible both premolars are perpendicularly oriented and the lateral incisor and canine are mesially angulated like both molars.

*For example: Kraus, B.S., Jordan, R.E., and Abrams, L., *Dental Anatomy and Occlusion.* (Baltimore: Williams & Wilkins, 1969).

The Permanent Dentition

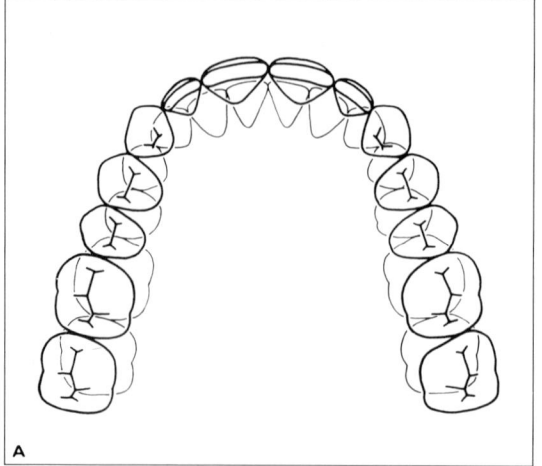
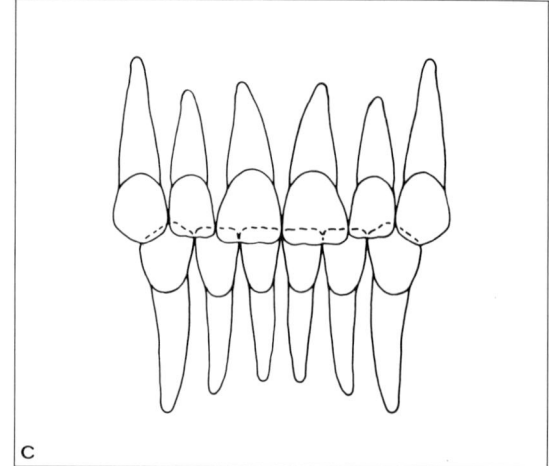
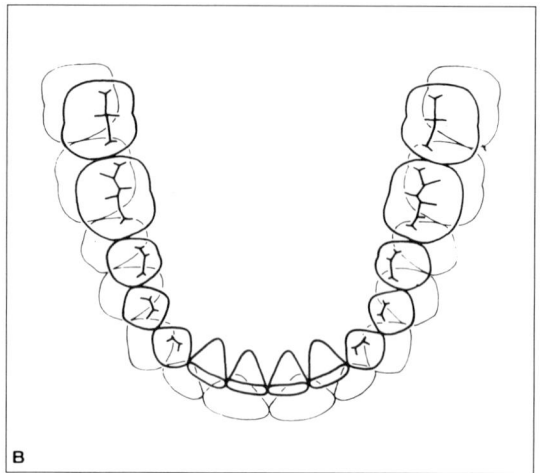
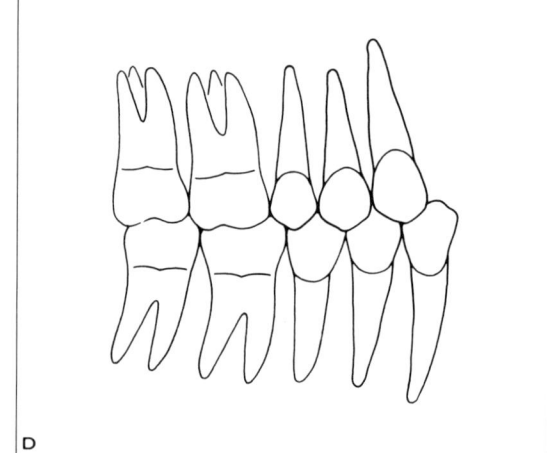

Figure 7-1

The mandibular molars are lingually inclined; the mandibular incisors slightly labially. In the maxilla the teeth in the posterior region are more or less buccally inclined; the incisors distinctly labially (Fig. 7-2).

The ideal inclination and angulation* of permanent teeth usually described in dental textbooks does not conform to the situation generally encountered in nature. [29] The ultimate location of the apices of the permanent teeth is determined primarily by the morphology of both jaws and by the spatial conditions within. The location of the

*In this work, the term *inclination* applies to the axial orientation of a tooth in labiolingual/buccolingual direction; the term *angulation* to the axial orientation in mesiodistal direction.

Fig. 7-1 Survey of the situation in the normal permanent dentition.

A   All adjacent maxillary teeth contact each other. Together, they form a harmoniously shaped dental arch. The maxillary teeth occlude slightly buccally with the mandibular ones. A small overjet is present in the incisor region.
B   All adjacent mandibular teeth contact each other as well and together form a harmoniously shaped dental arch on which the maxillary one fits. All mandibular teeth make contact with two opposing maxillary ones, with the exception of the mandibular central incisors.
C   The maxillary lateral incisors are shorter than the central ones, which in turn are exceeded in length by the canines. The incisal edges of the maxillary lateral incisors are slightly superior to those of the central ones and to the cusp tips of the canines. The roots of the maxillary lateral incisors are distally angulated, as are those of the central ones, but to a lesser extent. The incisal edges of the four mandibular incisors are in one plane. The cusp tips of the mandibular canines extend somewhat superiorly to that plane. The roots of the mandibular lateral incisors are slightly distally angulated. The mandibular lateral incisor is longer than the central one. The former, in turn, is shorter than the canine.
D   The canines and premolars intercuspate as do gear wheels. This is less the case for the permanent molars. The roots of the maxillary teeth are distally angulated with the exception of those of the second premolars; these are approximately perpendicularly oriented to the occlusal plane. The same applies to both mandibular premolars. The roots of the mandibular canines and molars are distally oriented.

crowns and the buccolingual inclination of the teeth are determined predominantly by the tongue and by the perioral musculature (the lips and cheeks). In this respect not only the length and volume of the soft tissue structures count, but also the positions occupied in a relaxed situation are essential. Moreover, the manner of function of these structures plays a role. In addition, other normal and abnormal functional aspects of the face are of importance. It has to be emphasized that the shape and size of the crowns of the teeth, the surrounding supporting tissues, the forces working within the dentition, and the way the masticatory system functions all are important factors in determining the individual tooth positions.[62]

The Permanent Dentition

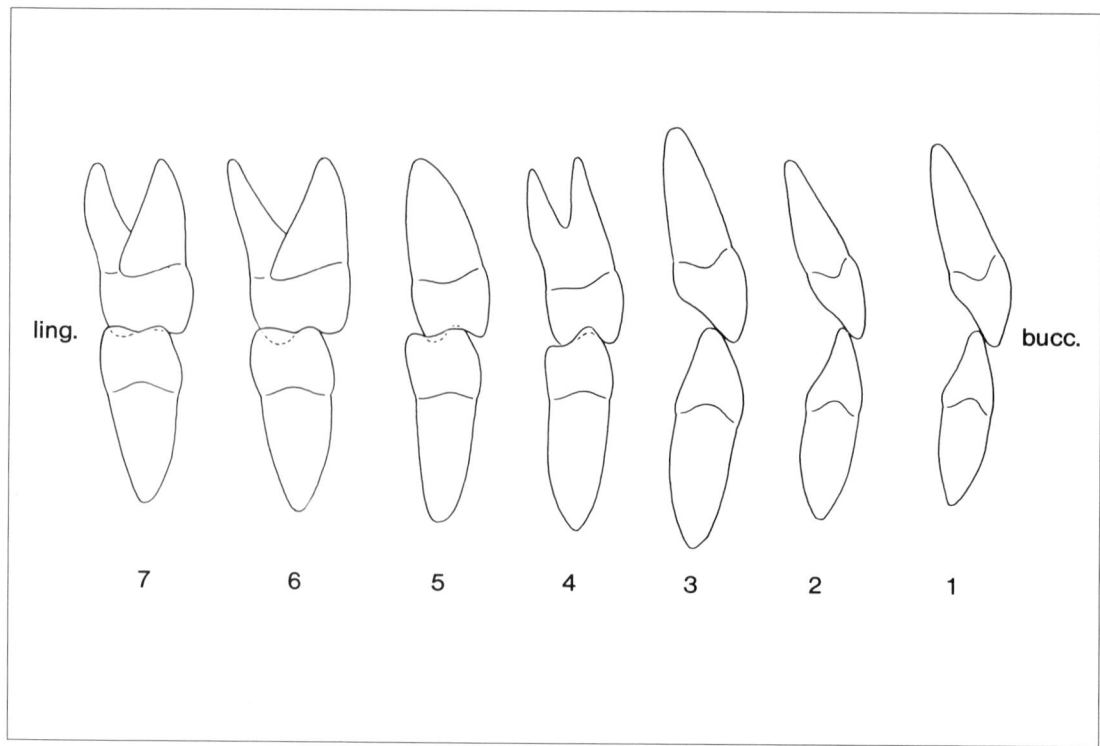

Fig. 7-2 Normal buccolingual inclination of the permanent teeth in both jaws. The corresponding maxillary and mandibular teeth are drawn in contact with each other. This does not conform to reality, as the contacts indicated here do not exist as such. Moreover, the mesial aspects of all teeth are shown instead of cross sections through the centers.
Both central incisors are labially inclined; the mandibular less, the maxillary more. The maxillary lateral incisor demonstrates the most distinct labial inclination of all teeth. The mandibular lateral incisor is more labially inclined than the adjacent central one. Also, both canines are buccally inclined, again more in the upper than in the lower jaw. Both maxillary premolars are buccally inclined. The mandibular ones are about perpendicularly oriented to the occlusal plane. The maxillary first and second permanent molars are buccally inclined; the mandibular ones lingually.
All maxillary teeth converge collectively in the cranial direction. This does not apply to the mandibular teeth. The mandibular incisors and canines are labially inclined, the mandibular molars lingually, with the premolars in between, defining reversal territory.

Finally, the statement is made that the occlusal relation between antagonists in the posterior regions is maintained by the contact that is established between both dental arches each time that the teeth are brought together. Normally, such a contact is made during every act of swallowing. An individual swallows 500 to 2,000 times in a 24-hour period.[52,74] Thus, the relation between the contacting posterior teeth is confirmed when habitual occlusion is established. In the maintenance of the position of the maxillary and mandibular incisors, the tongue and lips play a special role.

Chapter 8

Some General Aspects of the Normal Development of the Dentition

In the preceding chapters the development of the dentition has been presented in separate phases. Some aspects related to the overall development will be treated here. First, the changes taking place in the two dental arches and the alterations in their relation between birth and adulthood will be treated. Second, some facets of eruption will be discussed. Finally, a few general remarks regarding the development of the dentition will be made. The contents of this chapter entail that repetition of some features discussed earlier cannot be avoided.

The regions of the jaws containing the teeth prior to and after emergence do not increase gradually in size. Moreover, the increase in size of the different regions varies distinctly in amount and in timing. The sections of both jaws housing the deciduous dentition from the central incisors through the first deciduous molars grow considerably from birth to 6–8 months of age.[23] Thereafter, the increase is limited. The width of the dental arches increases only slightly as it is expressed by the limited enlargement of the transverse dimensions between the left and right deciduous canines. Between the first deciduous molars the increase is even smaller.[24,63,72,94] (See also Chapter 17.) A comparable limited increase takes place in the dental arch depth, measured as the distance from the labial surface of the central incisors to the center of the line connecting the distal surfaces of the first deciduous molars. The limited increase in dimensions of the sections of the dental arches discussed here is not restricted to the period of the development of the deciduous dentition. It also applies to the subsequent development to the adult stage.

The changes in transverse width and sagittal depth of the dental arches, occurring after the deciduous dentition has been completed, are primarily associated with processes accompanying the transitions. In both dental arches the increase in distance between the deciduous canines occurs mainly during the process of replacement of the incisors. The second spurt in intercanine distance increase is associated with the transition of the canines. The permanent canines attain a slightly more buccal position in the dental arch than their predecessors. The difference in this respect is more distinct for the maxillary than for the mandibular dental arch. Generally a gradual, continuous, and limited increase in the transverse dimension between corresponding left and right deciduous molars/premolars and permanent molars takes place from the complete deciduous dentition stage until the adult situation is reached. These increases in dental arch width dimensions are larger in the ventral region than in the dorsal region and the increases are smaller in the mandible than in the maxilla. This dissimilarity in increase in dental arch width dimension is associated with the more ventral displacement of the mandibular dental arch than of the maxillary one during normal development while the proper transverse relation between the opposing posterior teeth is maintained.

The discontinuous increases in dental arch width dimensions in the canine region, associated with the transitions, are superimposed on those that are more continuous in nature and correspond with comparable increases in dental arch width dimensions more posteriorly. The changes in the dental arches are illustrated in Figures 8-1 through 8-4. The left and right side drawings in these figures are essentially the same. The only dissimilarity is the thickness and continuity of lines and the presence of the occlusal patterns. In the drawings A and B in each figure, the earlier stage is accentuated; in drawings C and D, the later stage.

In both jaws the dental arch of the complete deciduous dentition describes a nearly flat occlusal plane. A vertical overbite (the overlap in height of the maxillary and mandibular incisors) is scarcely present. After the transition, the maxillary and mandibular permanent incisors erupt further than their predecessors were positioned. The result is a vertical overbite. An overlap of one-third of the clinical crown height* of the mandibular central incisor, measured perpendicularly to the occlusal plane, is considered normal in this respect. During the intertransitional period this overlap is usually slightly larger. This also holds true for the associated overjet. By overjet (sagittal overbite) is meant the distance between the labial side of the incisal edge of the maxillary central incisor and the labial surface of the mandibular central incisor measured parallel to the occlusal plane. In the second transitional period and thereafter, the maxillary and mandibular incisors start to upright. Their labial inclination reduces. The vertical and sagittal overbites become smaller.[13,14,35,51]

The permanent dentition does not have a flat occlusal plane, but one indicated by the term "curve of Spee." By this term is meant the imaginary curve that can be constructed through the buccal cusps and incisal edges of the teeth in a dental arch. Seen from the lateral side this curve is concave in the mandible. The mandibular molars and incisors are more superiorly positioned than the teeth in between. In the maxilla the situation is reversed. The curve of Spee is not present in the complete deciduous dentition; it develops during the first transitional period and stabilizes by adulthood.

The relatively dorsal position of the mandible in relation to the maxilla, initially present at birth, is caught up for the greater part during the first year of postnatal life. In this year the mandible demonstrates a larger ventral development than the maxilla. This process continues, albeit slightly, in the following years till facial growth is completed. Due to this slight dissimilarity in ventral development between the two jaws,

---

*The clinical crown height is the height of the visible tooth crown in the mouth.

Some General Aspects of Normal Development

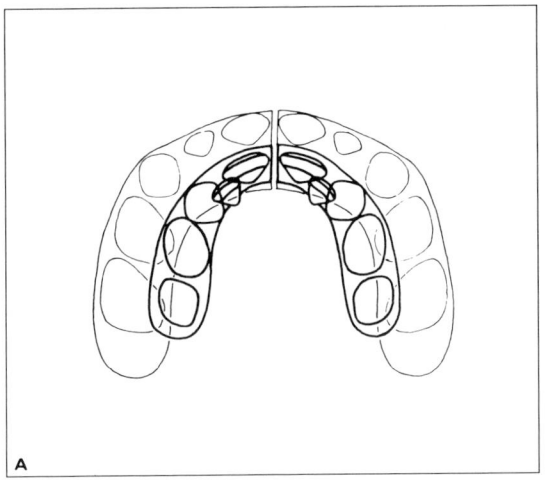
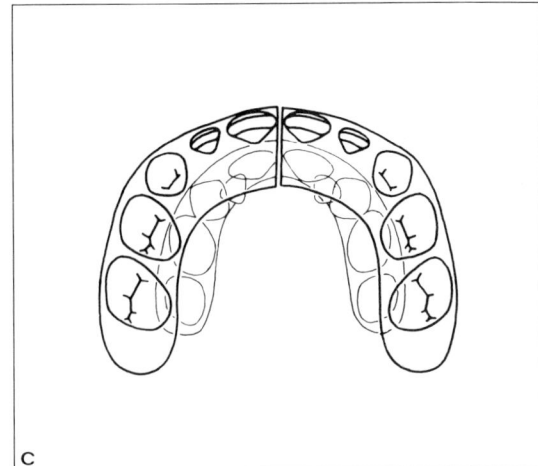
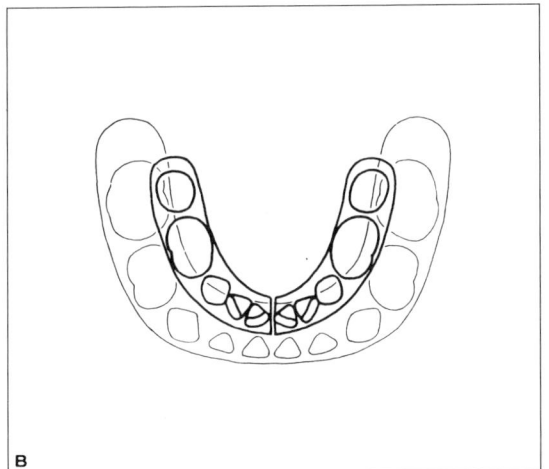
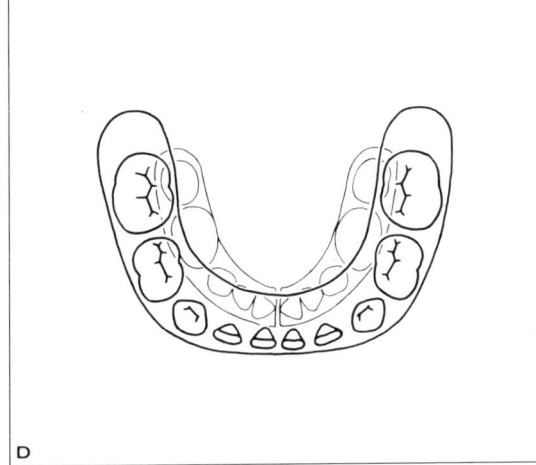

Fig. 8-1 Survey of the changes of the sections of the jaws containing the deciduous teeth, from birth to the complete deciduous dentition stage. During this period, the relevant sections of the jaws increase in size considerably. More than sufficient space develops for the deciduous incisors and canines. Substantial extension takes place in the dorsal direction. The increase in size of the anterior regions of the two dental arches takes place for the greater part during the first to eighth months after birth and before the mandibular symphysis begins to calcify. The median maxillary suture persists. In the maxilla, growth at the median plane can continue, in contrast with the situation in the mandible.

Some General Aspects of Normal Development

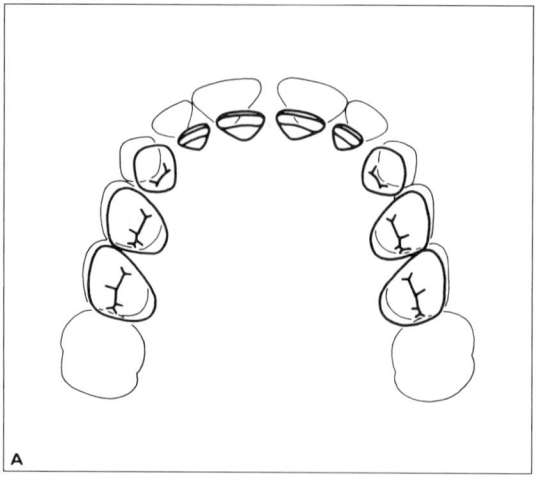

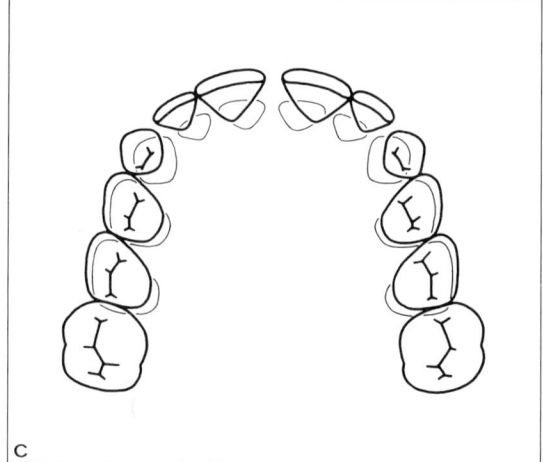

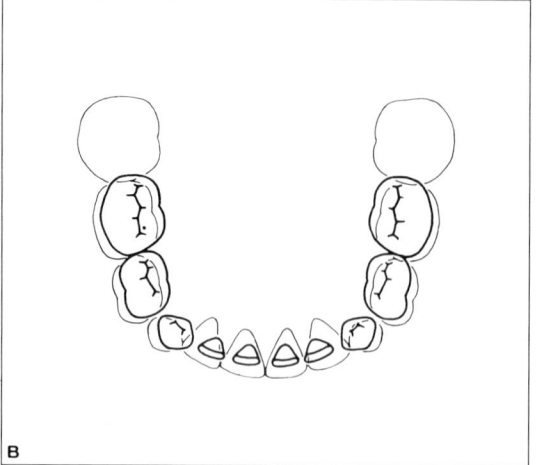

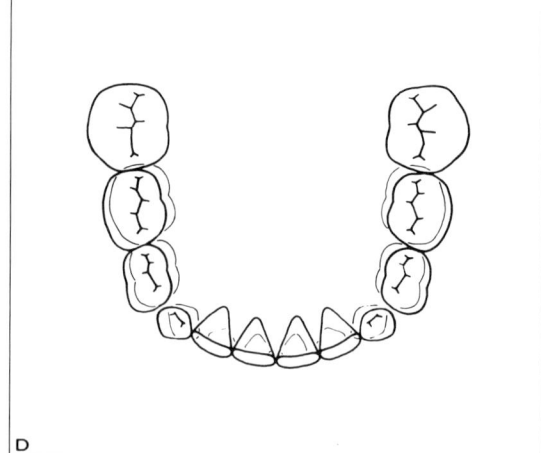

Fig. 8-2 Survey of the changes in both dental arches from the complete dentition stage to the intertransitional period.
The permanent incisors have arrived at a more ventral position than that of their predecessors. The intercanine distance has increased. The distance between the corresponding left and right deciduous molars has enlarged also, but more slightly. The first permanent molars have emerged dorsally to the dental arches. The diastemata in the posterior regions have been reduced. In each dental arch, the distal surfaces of the second deciduous molars have attained a more mesial position in relation to the canines.

Some General Aspects of Normal Development

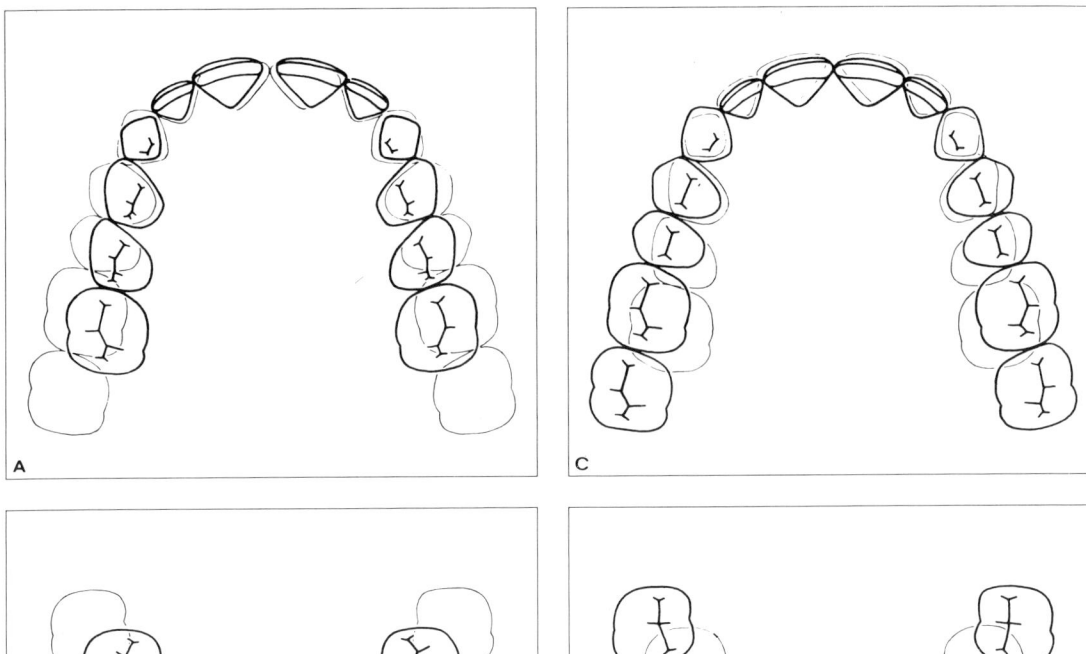

Fig. 8-3 Survey of the changes in both dental arches from the intertransitional period to the permanent dentition stage (with the exception of the third molars).
The canines have been replaced. The premolars are more buccally positioned than their predecessors were. The first permanent molars, and particularly the mandibular ones, have migrated mesially over some distance. The possibility for this mesial migration was supplied by the difference in mesiodistal crown dimensions between the deciduous molars and the premolars and the presence of diastemata in the dental arches. The second permanent molars have emerged dorsally to the dental arches.

Some General Aspects of Normal Development

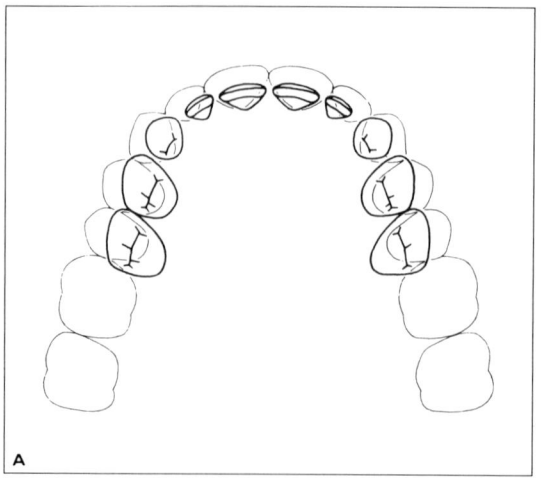
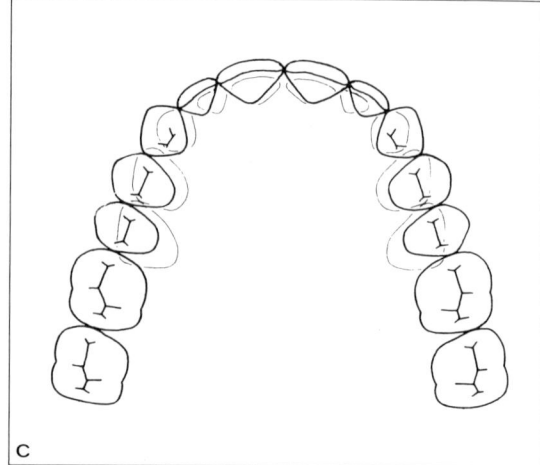
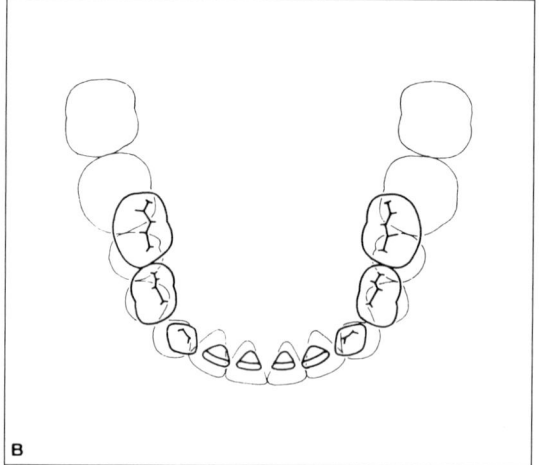
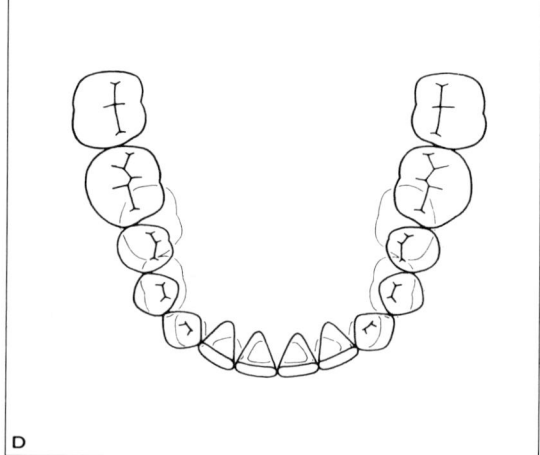

Fig. 8-4   Survey of the changes in both dental arches from the complete deciduous dentition stage to the permanent dentition stage (with the exception of the third molars).
The anterior sections of both dental arches increase only slightly in ventral and transverse dimensions. The transverse changes are more marked in the maxilla than in the mandible as the mandibular dental arch attains a more anterior position in relation to the maxillary one over time. The increase in size of both dental arches is achieved mainly by a dorsal extension. Successively, the first and the second permanent molars have been added to the dental arches. Harmonious emergence of the third molars will take place when it is preceded by sufficient extension of the jaws.

Some General Aspects of Normal Development

the sagittal relation between the two dental arches alters. The mandibular teeth gradually attain a more ventral position in relation to the maxillary ones. This phenomenon is partly responsible for the changes in occlusion of the first permanent molars, occurring in the passage of an end-to-end occlusion (flush terminal plane of the second deciduous molars), to a normal and solid intercuspation.[18,38] A good first permanent molar occlusion involves a more anterior position of the mesial surface of the mandibular first molar in relation to that of the maxillary first molar of one-half mesiodistal premolar crown width. In most cases the passage of an end-to-end relation of the first permanent molars to the proper relation is realized, for the greater part, through a more mesial migration of the mandibular first permanent molar than of the maxillary one. The possibility for this dissimilarity in mesial migration is supplied by the greater difference in mesiodistal crown dimensions between the deciduous molars and the premolars in the mandible than in the maxilla. In particular, the mandibular second deciduous molar is often extra wide in cases with a flush terminal plane (see Chapter 3).
A third factor of importance in the attainment of the ultimate molar occlusion is formed by the closure in mesial direction of the diastemata in the mandible. In particular, a large diastema between the first deciduous molar and canine (in which the maxillary deciduous canine occludes) can contribute to an improvement of the first permanent molar relation.[9]

The process of eruption of deciduous teeth differs from that of the permanent teeth, which are preceded by deciduous ones. In the newborn, the forming deciduous teeth are not covered by bone occlusally. Emergence is partly realized by "peeling" of the teeth and partly by an increase in the eruption rate. Unlike the deciduous molars, the permanent ones are initially covered by bone occlusally, and have a preemergence eruption phase. Subsequently, they emerge by a process comparable to the one described above for the deciduous molars. Also in that respect, the permanent molars correspond more with the deciduous teeth than the permanent ones do with their predecessors.
The premolars erupt through the path freed by resorption of the roots of the deciduous molars and of the interlying bone. No extra bone has to be removed for the passage of the premolar crowns, as is the case for permanent incisors and canines. Permanent incisors and canines do not emerge on the same surface as their predecessors, but slightly more lingually; moreover, they have larger crowns than their predecessors. A special and larger passage has to be prepared for emerging permanent incisor and canine crowns. The differences indicated here about processes associated with emergence between premolars and permanent incisors and canines are correlated with the differences between the two groups in the time that elapses between the loss of deciduous teeth and the emergence of their successors. This lapse of time is usually smaller for the canines than for the incisors. The interval is negative for deciduous molars and premolars, as the latter usually have already emerged prior to the shedding of the former (see Chapter 6).
Finally, the comment is made that a deciduous tooth at the very end of its presence in the oral cavity is no longer fixed by fibers connecting the tooth with the alveolar bone. Only the fibers running from the remaining part of the root to the gingiva keep the

Some General Aspects of Normal Development

tooth attached. This limited fixation of the tooth shortly before shedding allows the marked mobility then present. It further permits a deciduous tooth to attain a final position that deviates significantly from the location previously occupied in the dental arch.

Permanent teeth usually begin to erupt when their roots are formed to about one-quarter of the length that will ultimately be attained. Two to three years elapse before they subsequently reach the occlusal side of the bone of the covering alveolar process. At that stage two-thirds of the root are formed. After approximately half a year, the gingival tissue is perforated. Upon emergence, an initially rapid eruption follows. The occlusal half of the anatomical crown is visible after about four months. Eight months after emergence, about four-fifths of the height of the crown is uncovered.[15,32,33,39,71,76,91,100]

After an emerged tooth reaches its antagonist, the relation with the latter will determine the type of occlusal contact that will be attained. Usually the establishment of occlusal contact will be associated with changes in localization, inclination, and angulation. The roots are not yet formed completely. In general, the forming part of a tooth stays more or less in the same place. A displacement of a tooth associated with the establishment of occlusal contact will affect the relation between the already formed root and the tooth forming part. Deviations in root ends may result. These root end deviations can become reduced in later years by secondary cement deposition. Many adolescents and young adults have root end deviations that may cause complications in dental practice in the extraction of teeth.

The height levels on which the tooth forming parts initially (and also later) are located in relation to the occlusal plane are probably correlated with the tooth lengths ultimately to be attained (Fig. 8-5). The hypothesis is presented that differences in ultimate permanent tooth lengths—with the exception of the third molars—are related to differences in height levels of the formation of individual teeth. In accordance with this hypothesis is the observation that permanent canines, which will end up as the longest teeth, are formed at the farthest distance from the occlusal plane. Further, the ultimately rather short maxillary lateral incisors are formed nearer the occlusal plane than the central ones, which will attain a longer tooth length. The situation illustrated in Figure 8-5 is the most common one. However, a certain variation exists in this respect.

The time of beginning of calcification of the individual teeth within the jaws differs markedly. The second permanent molar begins its calcification considerably later than the first one; the same applies to the third in relation to the second. Further, the second permanent molar emerges approximately six years later than the first one. The third one also follows the second after approximately six years. However, the levels at which the roots of the first and the second molar are formed are at about the same height in each jaw. The root ends of an almost completely formed first permanent molar are directly adjacent to the forming part of the second molar furcation, which is under development (compare Fig. 5-1). The mandibular third molar is initially formed in the vertical part of the mandible and located more superiorly. The calcification of its cusp tips starts at about the level of the occlusal plane.

Some General Aspects of Normal Development

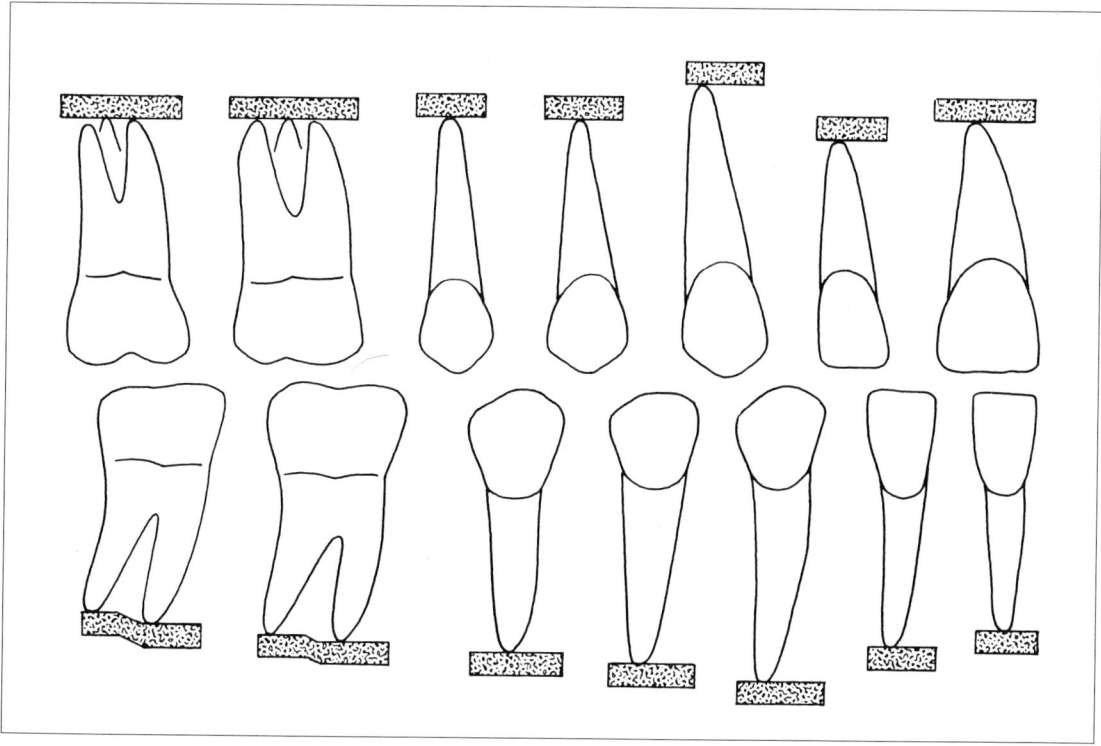

Fig. 8-5 Survey of the assumed relation between the length of permanent teeth ultimately to be attained and the height levels of formation.
The level of initial tooth formation is shaded. The maxillary canine is formed adjacent to the piriform aperture and farther away from the occlusal plane than any other tooth. The maxillary canine becomes the longest tooth. The maxillary central incisor is formed in close proximity to the nasal floor and is initially farther away from the occlusal plane than is the lateral incisor. Also, in the mandible, the formation of the canine is at the greatest distance from the occlusal plane. The formation of the lateral incisor is nearer to the occlusal plane, and that holds even more true for the central incisor. The ultimate variation in tooth length follows accordingly.

Subsequently the mandibular third molar gradually attains a more inferior position as the other teeth continue their vertical displacement. In the maxilla the third molar is formed more cranially in the region of the maxillary tuberosity than the second permanent molar.

Deciduous teeth are approximately perpendicularly oriented in relation to the occlusal plane. This applies to the buccolingual inclination as well as to the mesiodistal angulation. In some sense this perpendicular orientation partly accounts for the location of the permanent incisors and canines lingually to the roots of their predecessors. The forming premolars are situated between the roots of their predecessors. Deciduous molars have markedly diverging roots and a furcation in close proximity to the crown.

Typical for the regions of the deciduous molars and the first permanent molars is the absence of crowding in a normally developing dentition. The reverse applies to the maxillary second and third permanent molars. The region of the maxilla in which these teeth are formed has not attained its ultimate size by the time the crowns have been formed. In this respect the formation of the teeth runs ahead of the growth of the jaw in the maxillary tuberosity regions. The forming maxillary second and third permanent molars are oriented distobuccally with their occlusal surfaces. The further these teeth are formed and descend, the more their orientation changes. However, at emergence the distal angulation and buccal inclination are still present, although in reduced form. Not until all permanent teeth in the maxillary molar region have erupted fully and have attained occlusion can the changes in orientation leading to a normal angulation and inclination start to take place.

In the meantime, additional growth at the tuberosity region has contributed slightly to the space that earlier was too small to house the maxillary second and third permanent molar crowns harmoniously. Moreover, the roots of the maxillary second and third molars are smaller in diameter than their crowns. Hence, upon complete eruption the roots have ample space and the teeth can attain the correct angulation and inclination.

The situation in the mandible is different. The mandibular permanent molars are initially formed in the region of the jaw where the horizontal part meets the vertical part. During their development, the permanent molars are positioned more posteriorly in the mandible than their crowns will be located after occlusion has been attained years later. In transverse direction, the crowns are initially formed in the area where later the roots will be positioned. This area is more buccally located than where the occlusal surfaces will be situated after occlusion has been attained. No crowding exists as it does in the corresponding area of the maxilla. Problems in the mandibular molar region do not appear unless the horizontal part of the jaw containing the dentition increases insufficiently. Then the last mandibular permanent molar cannot attain a more upright position and emerge without problems.

In the anterior part of both jaws the deciduous as well as the permanent incisors and canines are formed in a situation of crowding as explained before. Preceding the emergence of the deciduous dentition, the growth of both jaws is so large that the teeth can align and attain a harmonious position before appearing in the oral cavity.

Some General Aspects of Normal Development

This is not the case for the permanent incisors and canines because the growth of the jaws required for that purpose is not realized. Moreover, if such an extensive growth took place, both jaws would become so large that diastemata might develop and could be maintained. The permanent incisors would not become labially inclined, but become positioned more or less perpendicularly in the jaws, as the deciduous incisors were.

The absence of spontaneous correction of the crowded positions of the mandibular and maxillary permanent incisors prior to emergence is related to the phenomenon that those teeth develop in a region not suited for the temporary housing of the crowns, but designed to contain only the smaller roots later. Consequently, the transition of the mandibular and particularly the maxillary incisors is associated with a temporary positioning of the permanent teeth that appears unharmonious when compared with the ideal adult situation. Nevertheless, this situation has to be considered normal and typical for a harmonious development of the dentition. Interference in this normal process is undesirable.

The development of the dentition deviates markedly from that of other parts and structures of the body. Crowns of teeth are formed directly to their ultimate size and are housed within the jaws for years before they can emerge. Furthermore, the jaws have to contain not only the roots of the deciduous teeth, but also the partly formed and relatively large permanent teeth at the same time. In some regions, such as the maxillary incisor one, this agglomerate of deciduous and permanent teeth is packed in a space that later only has to contain the roots of the permanent teeth with relatively small diameters.

In studying the development of the dentition, one becomes impressed by the intricacy of the different processes involved and by the ingenious way in which these processes interplay. The complexity of the development of the dentition becomes even more intriguing when it is realized that it takes place within the confines of the growth of the face, which in itself is not a simple process either. It is not easy to disclose the secrets of the development of the dentition. However, it will be easier to understand the ingenious way in which many processes take place if one tries to detect and understand the relations and interactions between the different phenomena involved.

Chapter 9

Abnormalities in the Dental Arches

A number of abnormalities that may occur in the dental arches are treated in this chapter. These abnormalities are not discussed in terms of their developmental characteristics. This treatise is restricted to the description of various deviations in the dental arches, supported by systematic drawings.
In view of the intricate processes typical for the development of the dentition, the occurrence of abnormalities in the dental arches is not astonishing. On the contrary, it is amazing that the developmental processes so often come to a good end and that relatively few deviations evolve.
The most frequently occurring abnormality in the dental arches is a discrepancy between the needed and the available dental arch perimeter. Such a discrepancy means that the space available for the teeth within a dental arch is either too small or too large to contain all teeth harmoniously and in contact with each other. These incongruities are indicated by the term "Arch Length Discrepancy" (ALD). This term leaves undecided whether the incongruity is caused by an excess of one component or a shortage of the other. The same applies to the terms "crowding" and "spacing".*
Crowding rarely occurs in the complete deciduous dentition, but appears frequently in later phases of the development of the dentition. In particular, crowding in the mandibular incisor canine region is rather common in the adult dentition.
Spacing is normally present in the deciduous dentition but rather infrequently in the permanent one. In the latter, it occurs primarily in the maxillary incisor canine region. Specifically, space in the median plane in the permanent dentition (a central diastema) is often perceived as disturbing.

Concerning the individual teeth, abnormalities in the development of the dentiton can be categorized as deviations in number, size, shape, and position.
Either too many or too few teeth can be formed. Deviations in the number of

*The term *Arch Length Discrepancy* is preferred over the term *Arch Length Deficiency*. The latter only applies to crowding; the former applies to both crowding (−value) and spacing (+value).

teeth in the deciduous dentition are rare; they are regularly encountered in the permanent dentition. Absence of teeth based on nonformation (agenesis) occurs quite often. The sequence of diminishing frequency in agenesis is[3]: third molars (16%), the mandibular second premolars (4.4%), the maxillary lateral incisors (1.7%), and the maxillary second premolars (1.6%). Formation of other permanent teeth can fail (see Fig. 9-1) and more than one tooth can be missing in one individual (multiple agenesis). For statistical information on agenesis and other topics presented here, refer to Chapter 17.

Supernumerary teeth can be encountered everywhere in the dental arches and particularly in the mandibular and maxillary incisor regions. Most frequently, a supernumerary tooth occurs between the two maxillary central incisors adjacent to the median maxillary suture (mesiodens). Such a tooth often deviates in size and shape and can be oriented in all possible directions. Mesiodentes can be present two-fold or plural (Fig. 9-2).

Deviations in size are mostly of a relative nature. All teeth combined can appear either too large or too small in comparison with the size of the head and, specifically, the jaws. A relative excess of tooth material expresses itself either as crowding or as a marked dominance of the dentition (Double Protrusion [DP] of the maxillary and mandibular incisors) or a combination of both. With a relative shortage of tooth material the consequence will be either spacing in the dental arches or a retruded position of the incisors with the associated retroposition of the lips in relation to the chin and nose (dished-in profile), or a combination of both.

Deviations in the size of the individual teeth most frequently affect the maxillary lateral permanent incisors, appearing as undersized crowns. A deviation in mesiodistal crown dimension of one or more teeth in one dental arch—with the absence of corresponding and compensatory crown size differences in the opposing dental arch—will result in a disturbance in matching of the two dental arches without spacing or crowding.[16,17] This phenomenon is described as Tooth Size Discrepancy (TSD); some examples are presented in Figure 9-3.

Deviations in the shape of teeth usually present few problems. An exception in this respect is formed by the maxillary incisors. The laterals, in particular, rather often have abnormal crown shapes. Their crowns can be cone-shaped ("peg-shaped laterals") or have deviations of other forms. Moreover, oversized labiolingual crown dimensions of all four maxillary incisors, and specifically the central ones, can lead to deviations of the normal occlusion in the incisor region.

Deviations in the individual position of teeth occur very often. Teeth can be located too far away from the occlusal plane (infraposition) or they can be overerupted (supraposition). Deviations in axial orientation can happen in different directions. The same applies in regard to the position of individual teeth in relation to the other ones. A survey of deviating tooth positions and rotations with the related terminology is presented in Figures 9-4 and 9-5.

A special category of deviations in tooth positions is the one caused by ankylosis, a bony union between the cementum of the root and the adjacent bone of the alveolar socket. An ankylosed tooth cannot erupt any more and hence stays behind in the vertical development of the dentition. Occlusal contact is lost. The ankylosed tooth

Abnormalities in the Dental Arches

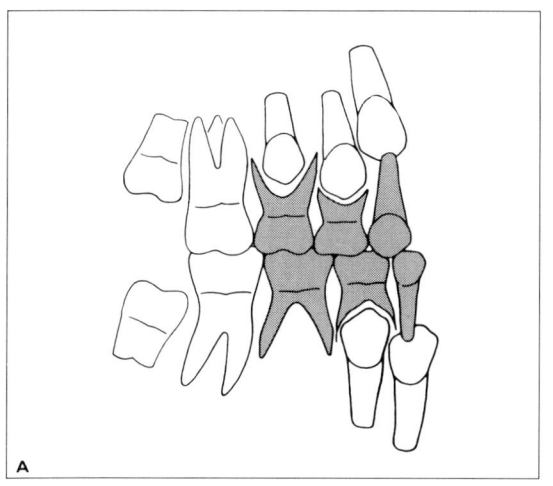
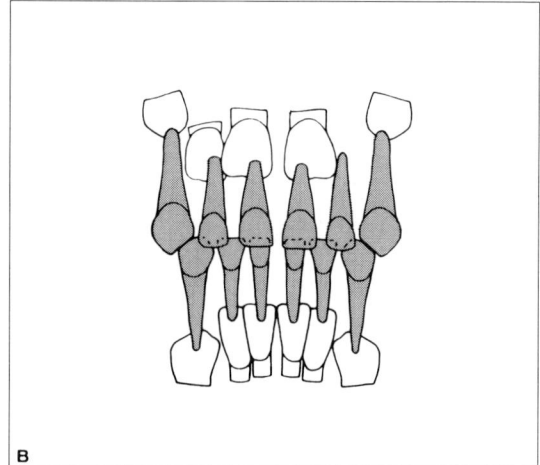
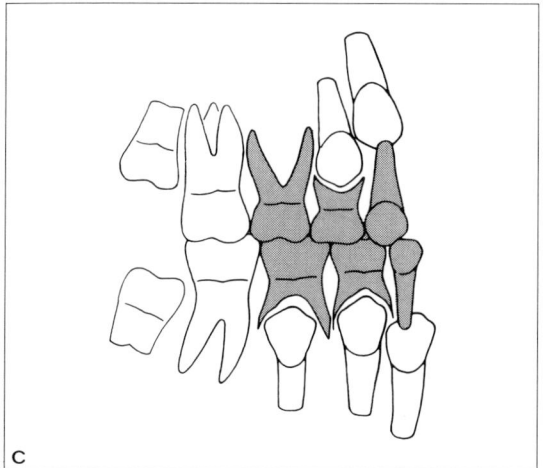
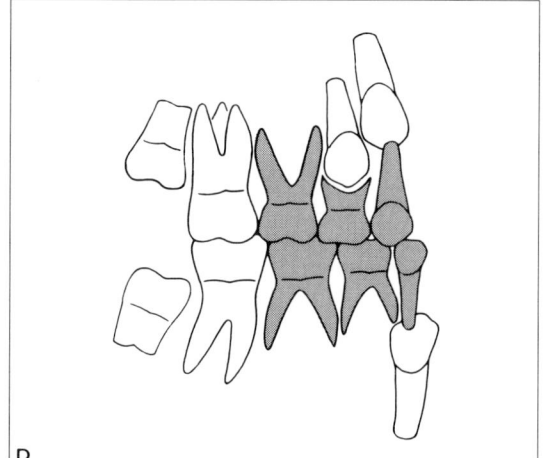

Fig. 9-1 Examples of the absence of teeth because of nonformation (agenesis).

A The third molar (16%) is most frequently not formed; next the mandibular second premolar (4.4%).
B The maxillary lateral incisor is the tooth most frequently not formed in the maxilla (1.7%).
C The maxillary second premolar is occasionally missing (1.6%).
D An example of multiple agenesis.

Abnormalities in the Dental Arches

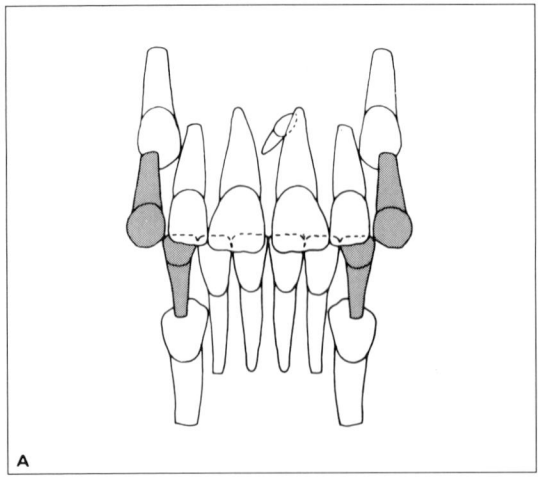
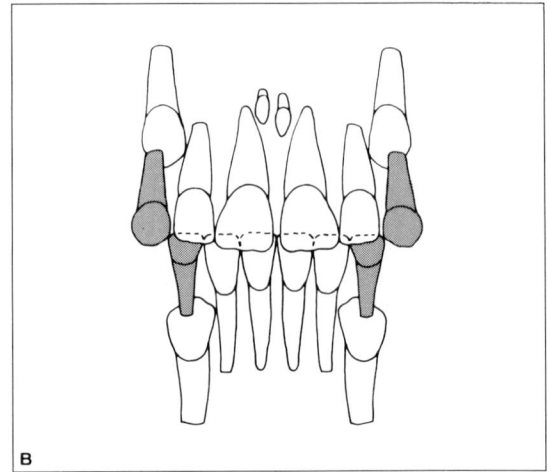
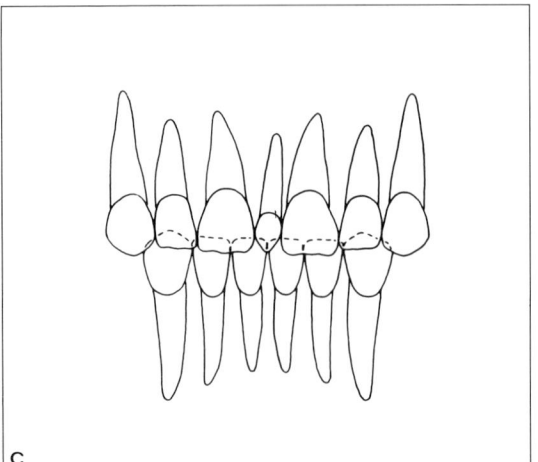
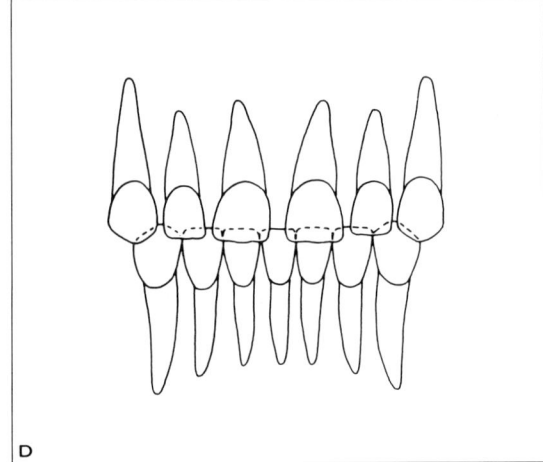

Fig 9-2 Examples of the occurrence of supernumerary teeth in the maxillary incisor region near the median plane (mesiodens) and of an extra incisor in the mandible.

A   A mesiodens of small size and cone shape positioned partially palatally to the maxillary left central permanent incisor.
B   Two mesiodentes.
C   A normally erupted extra maxillary central incisor, which is small in size and deviating in shape.
D   An anterior mandibular segment with five permanent incisors, all of normal size and shape.

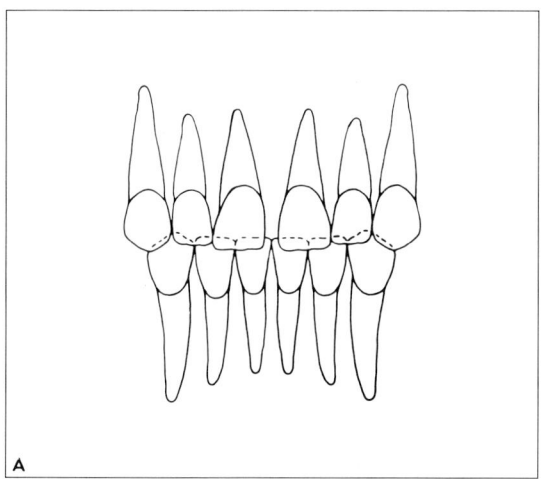
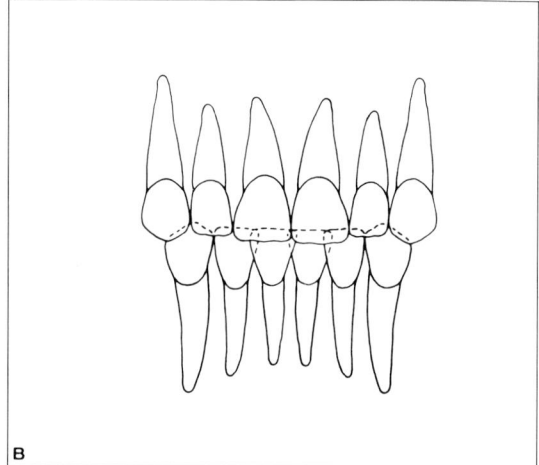
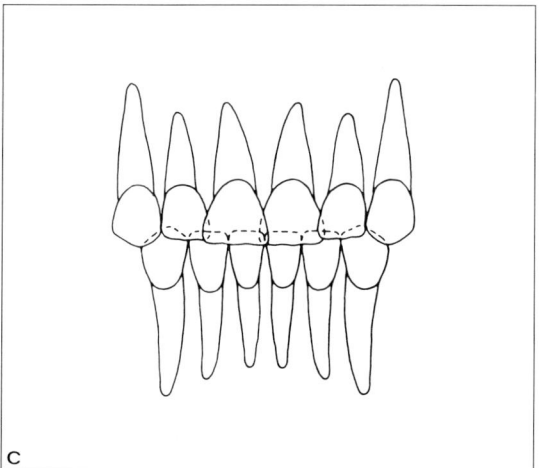
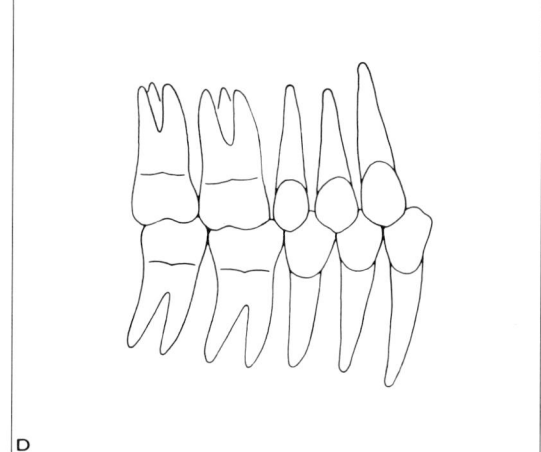

Fig. 9-3   Examples of Tooth Size Discrepancy (TSD).

A   Maxillary central incisors with relatively small mesiodistal crown dimensions, associated with a central diastema. The picture is the same when the mandibular incisor crowns are relatively too wide.
B   Crowding of the mandibular incisors with mesiodistal crown dimensions relatively too large to match harmoniously with their antagonists.
C   Relatively too wide maxillary incisor crowns with overlap of these teeth.
D   Lack of good contacts in the maxillary dental arch associated with maxillary premolars whose mesiodistal crown dimensions are too small in relation to those of their antagonists.

Abnormalities in the Dental Arches

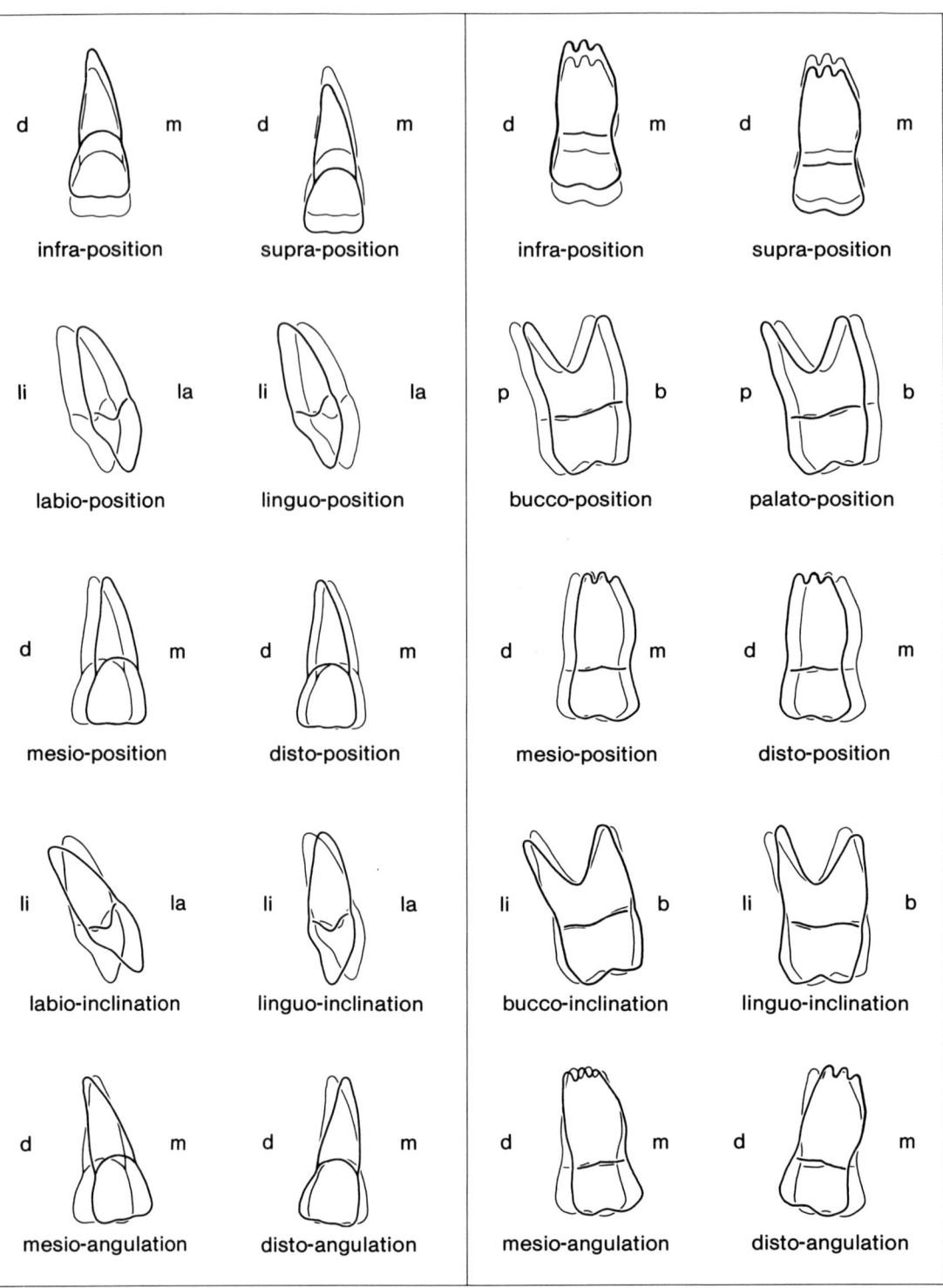

Figure 9-4

Abnormalities in the Dental Arches

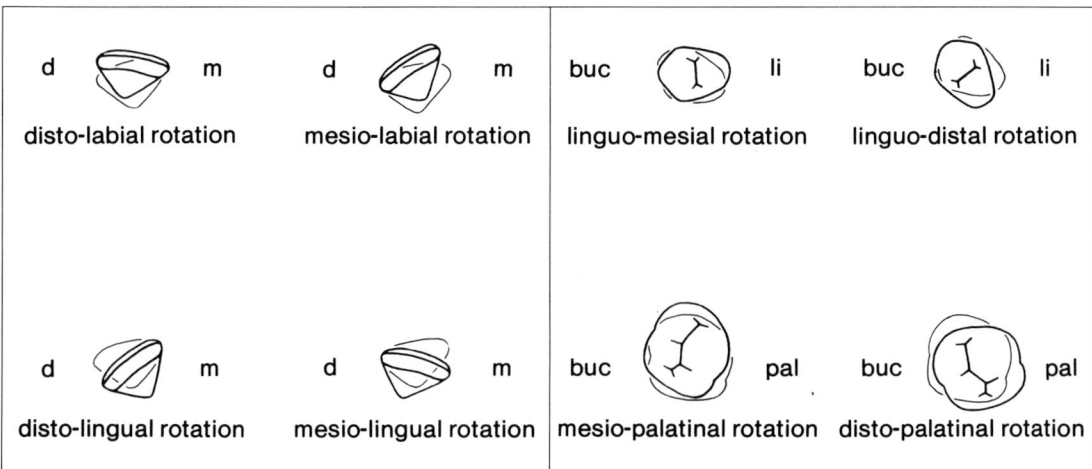

Fig. 9-5 Survey of some rotations of a maxillary right central incisor, a first premolar, and a first permanent molar. For the description of the rotations, the deviation of the crown is used as reference.

Fig. 9-4 Survey of deviating positions of teeth with the descriptive terms presented for the maxillary right central incisor and for the maxillary right first permanent molar. The normal situation is drawn with a thin line; the deviating position with a heavy one. The same applies to Figure 9-5. For the other maxillary teeth and for the mandibular ones the same descriptions are used for deviating positions and rotations. (For corresponding terms used to indicate the illustrated deviations, refer to Table 9-1.)
In the maxilla, the lingual surface is often referred to as the palatal.

77

becomes "submerged" as its neighbors continue to erupt. Ankylosis most frequently happens in mandibular deciduous molars. However, it also occurs in permanent teeth (Fig. 9-6). The size of the bony union present in an ankylosed tooth between the root surface and the alveolar socket can vary. Often the ankylosed area is limited in size. Little is known about the causes of this deviation, but it is assumed that traumata can lead to ankylosis.

Finally, two categories of the phenomenon of tooth impaction can be distinguished. The first is composed of teeth that can erupt, but do not; the second of teeth that try to erupt but cannot do so. To the first category belong teeth that do not start to erupt, while in the meantime their roots continue to be formed. The associated normal displacement toward the occlusal plane does not take place. Impacted teeth of this category are often abnormally positioned within the jaws (see Chapter 15). A partially erupted tooth, for example a maxillary permanent central incisor, can become displaced by a sudden dislocation of its predecessor. Eruption does not continue further; the tooth is impacted. The maxillary permanent canine is the most frequently impacted tooth in this category. The variation in position of impacted maxillary canines is large. The root of the preceding deciduous canine usually resorb only partially and can be maintained for years. Moreover, impaction can be caused by trauma (see Chapter 15).

The second category consists of teeth that are confronted with an obstacle in their eruption process. These teeth become impacted after their eruption has been partially realized. The most common cause for the arrest in eruption is lack of space. A classical example in this respect is the mandibular third molar retention in cases of insufficient mandibular growth to accommodate these teeth dorsally to the dental arches. Another example is the retention of a mandibular second premolar following a marked displacement and approximation of the adjacent permanent teeth because of premature loss of its predecessor.

In principle, all abnormalities in the dental arches discussed above can occur in all possible relations between the two dental arches. As such, they can be thought of as being superimposed on the deviations between both dental arches, which will be dealt with in subsequent chapters.

An incomplete list of terms to indicate deviations in the positions of individual teeth and in their mutual relations is found in Table 9-1. In evaluating these terms, it should be realized that sometimes a slight difference exists in the meaning of the terms arranged as equivalents. Moreover, not all authors use the same term for the same meaning.

Abnormalities in the Dental Arches

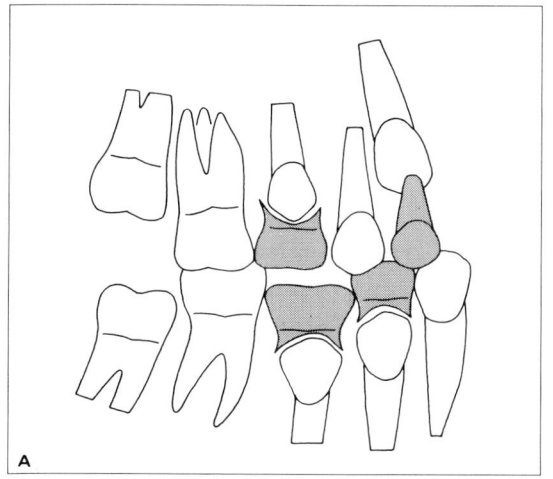 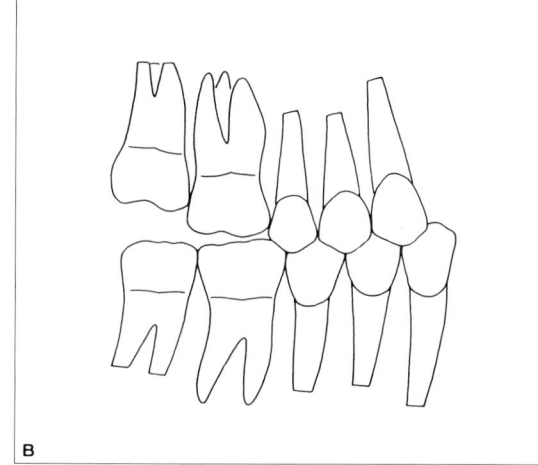

Fig. 9-6. Survey of two examples of ankylosed teeth.

A The mandibular second deciduous molar has become ankylosed and has remained behind in eruption, resulting in its submerged position. The resorption of the deciduous roots associated with the eruption of the succeeding premolar is usually normal but delayed. The roots of the deciduous molar, and the interlying bone, including the ankylosed area, continue to resorb.

B The maxillary first and second permanent molars are ankylosed. They erupted to a certain level until bony unions arose between the cementum and the alveolar sockets.

Table 9-1 Terms with equivalent meaning

Labioinclination, proclination, protrusion, labioversion, eversion
Linguoinclination, palatoinclination, retroinclination, retrusion, linguoversion, palatoversion, retroversion
Labioposition, proposition, protrusion
Linguoposition, palatoposition, retroposition, retrusion
Horizontal overbite, sagittal overbite, overjet
Vertical overbite, overbite
Class I occlusion, neutro-occlusion
Class II occlusion, disto-occlusion, postnormal occlusion
Class III occlusion, mesio-occlusion, prenormal occlusion

Chapter 10

The Development of the Dentition in Class II/1 Malocclusions

At the end of the last century, Dr. Edward H. Angle[1] introduced a classification of sagittal (anteroposterior) relations between the mandibular and maxillary dental arches. This classification is internationally accepted and was named after its inventor. The Angle Classification is still used commonly today.
The normal sagittal relation between the two dental arches is indicated with the term *Class I*. A dorsal position of the mandibular dental arch in relation to the maxillary one is specified as a *Class II malocclusion*. A reversed situation, with the mandibular dental arch too much ventrally in relation to the maxillary one, is called a *Class III malocclusion*. The terms Class II and Class III leave undecided whether the deviating component is located in the mandible or in the maxilla or in a combination of both. Only the sagittal relation between the two dental arches is indicated. No judgment is passed on causal factors. Later, the sagittal relation between the bony parts of the lower and upper jaws was added to the Angle Classification.[2] However, this aspect is not incorporated in this discussion nor in that of Class III malocclusions in Chapter 12.
Angle has further divided the Class II malocclusions into Class II division 1 (II/1) and Class II division 2 (II/2) malocclusions. In Class II/1 malocclusions, the maxillary incisors have a more or less normal labiolingual inclination or are too much protruded. In Class II/2 malocclusions, to be discussed separately in the next chapter, two or more maxillary incisors are tipped palatally. As the position of the lips is directly related to those of the incisors, a Class II/1 malocclusion may be associated with a lower lip situated between the mandibular and maxillary incisors. An adequate lip seal may not exist, particularly in children. In Class II/2 malocclusions, the lips are in contact with each other.
Sagittal deviations between the two dental arches, complicated by an asymmetry of the dental arch relation, have been labeled by Angle with the supplementary term subdivision. A Class II subdivision stands for a Class II dental arch relation on the one side and a Class I on the other side. The Class II/1 subdivision will not be dealt with here but will be treated together with the Class III subdivision in Chapter 14.

Abnormalities in the dental arches themselves, which may complicate a Class II/1 malocclusion, are not discussed in this chapter either. In principle, all abnormalities in the dental arches presented in chapter 9 can occur in Class I, Class II, and Class III conditions and may, as such, be thought of as superimposed on the sagittal dental arch relation.

In this discussion of Class II/1 malocclusions, basically normal conditions are assumed to be present in each dental arch. However, certain deviations in the location of maxillary and mandibular teeth are caused by the abnormal relation between the two dental arches. These deviations are exclusively the consequences of the abnormal sagittal relation and will be discussed in that context.

The Class II/1 malocclusions in the deciduous dentition (Fig. 10-1), in the intertransitional period (Fig. 10-2), and in the permanent dentition (Fig. 10-3) are described successively. In addition, the eruption of the first permanent molars and the transition of the incisors are treated (Figs. 10-4 and 10-5). Finally, the transition of the posterior teeth is discussed (Fig. 10-6).

A Class II/1 malocclusion without additional complications has a mandibular dental arch that conforms in shape to that of a Class I situation viewed occlusally. The mandibular dental arch in relation to the maxillary one is more dorsally positioned than in a Class I situation. Nevertheless, the transverse relation between the occluding posterior teeth has also been achieved through the cone-funnel mechanism upon attainment of initial contact. The established transverse relation of the posterior teeth is confirmed repeatedly each time the mandibular and maxillary dental arches touch in maximal occlusion. Within the lower jaw, little play exists in the location of the posterior teeth in the transverse direction. The bony structures containing the roots are limited in their labiolingual dimensions. In the maxilla, a larger variation exists in the location of the roots of the posterior teeth. The surrounding bony structures develop primarily owing to the presence of the locally erupting and subsequently functioning teeth.

In the maxilla, the location of the roots is not labially and lingually restricted by a heavy, thick wall of compact bone, as is the case in the lower jaw. In the mandible, compact bone is continuous around the inferior border and serves as a reinforcement. In contrast with the maxilla, the mandible is not attached to other bony structures and requires sufficient strength and body of its own. The mandible has to be robust enough to resist the forces of mastication and external powers exerted on it. In the maxilla, the forces of mastication are transmitted superiorly through adjacent structures to the calvarium. The mandible acts independently in this respect and has to cope with the forces of mastication on its own.[92] As has been explained before, at the end of the first year of postnatal life, the mandibular symphysis has calcified and the potency of transverse enlargement in the median plane of the lower jaw has been lost. However, in the maxilla the possibility for broadening is maintained as the maxillary median suture does not unite and preserves the potency for interstitial growth until the development of the dentition is completed. Consequently, the mandibular dental arch will function as a mold for the placement of the maxillary posterior teeth in transverse direction in the development

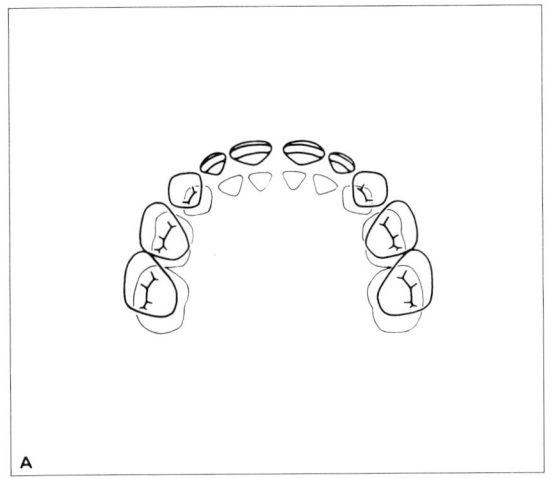
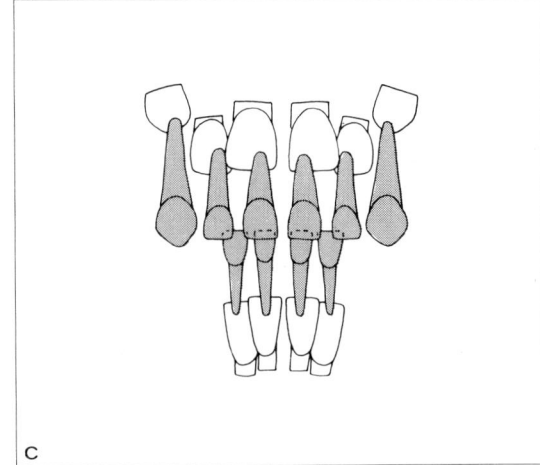
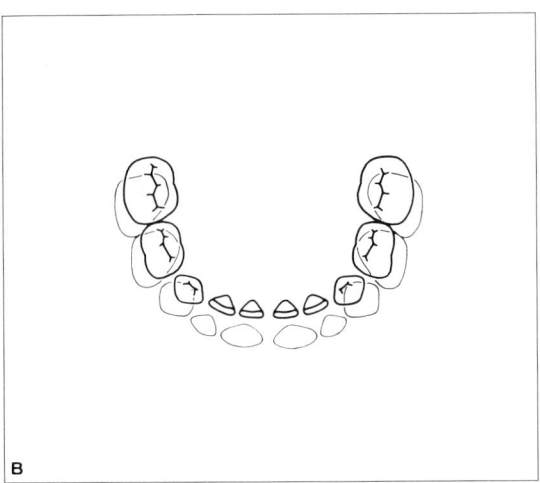
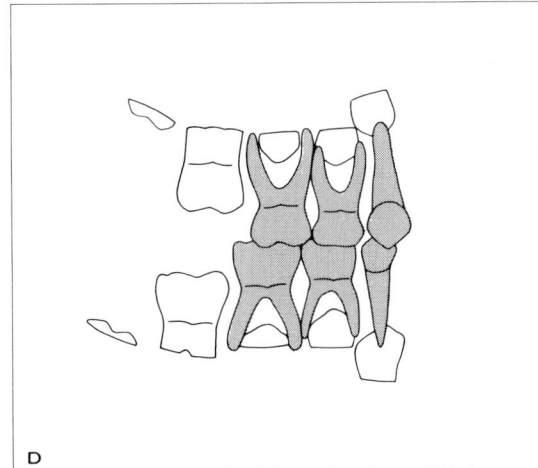

Fig. 10-1 Survey of a Class II/1 malocclusion in the complete deciduous dentition (compare with Fig. 3-1).

A,B The mandibular dental arch is dorsally situated in relation to the maxillary one. A good transverse relation exists between the opposing deciduous molars. The transverse dimensions of the mandibular dental arch are normal; those of the maxillary are too small.
C Limited increase of the overbite. The deciduous incisors usually do not overerupt until vertical support is attained. Otherwise, the overbite would have been larger (see also Fig. 10-5).
D In occlusion, the mandibular deciduous molars are positioned too far dorsally in relation to the maxillary ones. The terminal plane of the deciduous dentition exhibits a distal step.

Development in Class II/1 Malocclusions

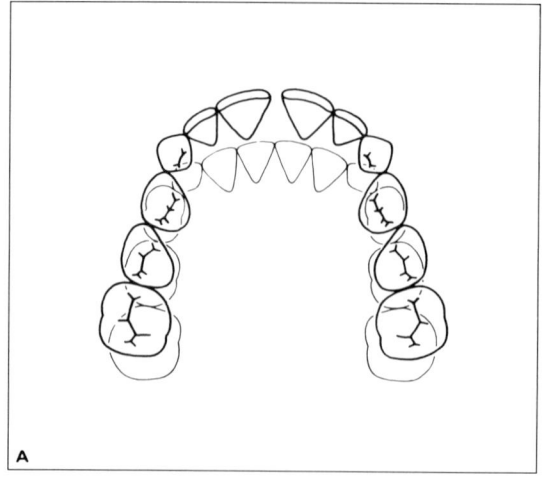
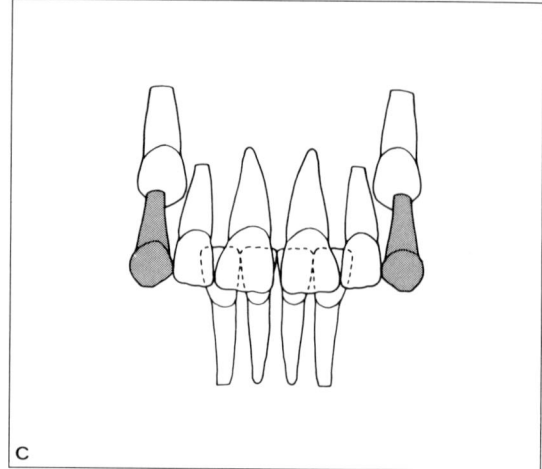
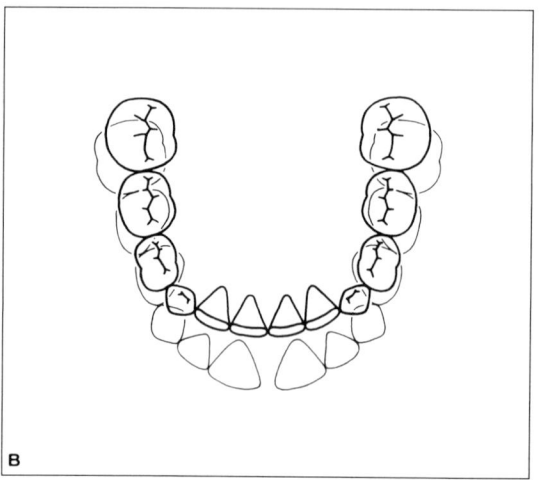
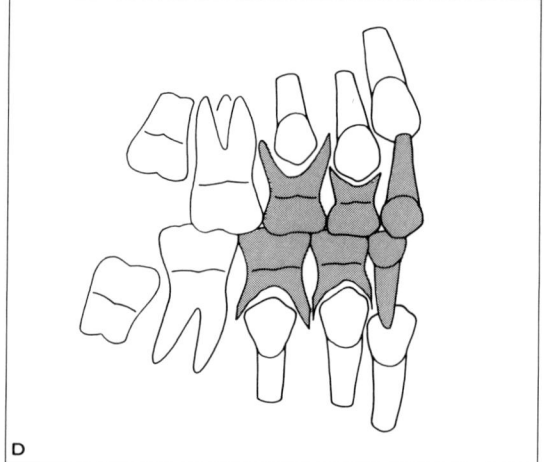

Fig. 10-2 Survey of a Class II/1 malocclusion in the intertransitional period (compare with Fig. 5-1).

A,B Dorsal position of the mandibular dental arch in relation to the maxillary one, abnormally large overjet, and a normal transverse relation between the opposing posterior teeth. Relatively too narrow and too tapering maxillary dental arch.

C Increased overbite. The permanent incisors erupt until vertical support is obtained in habitual occlusion. The incisal edges of the mandibular incisors may touch the palate instead of the lingual surfaces of the opposing teeth.

D The mandibular first permanent molar occludes too far dorsally to the maxillary one. However, the opposing surfaces of both teeth are quite large, as is the intercuspating area.

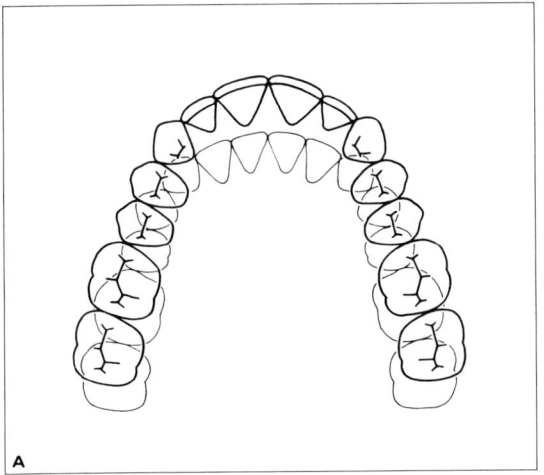 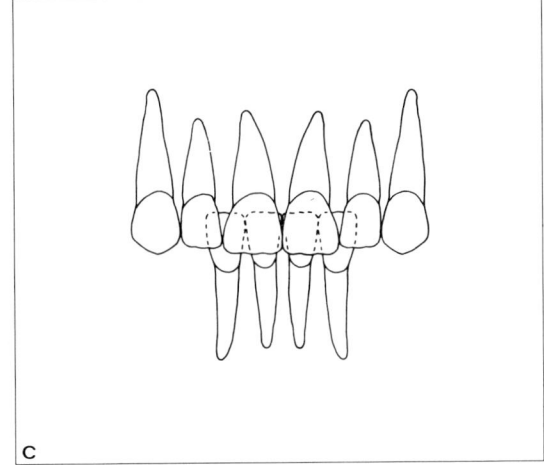
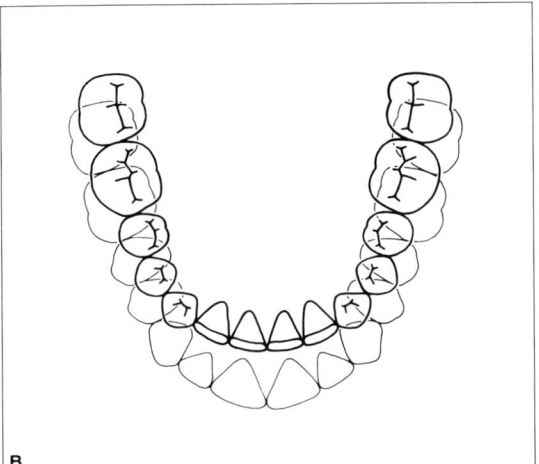 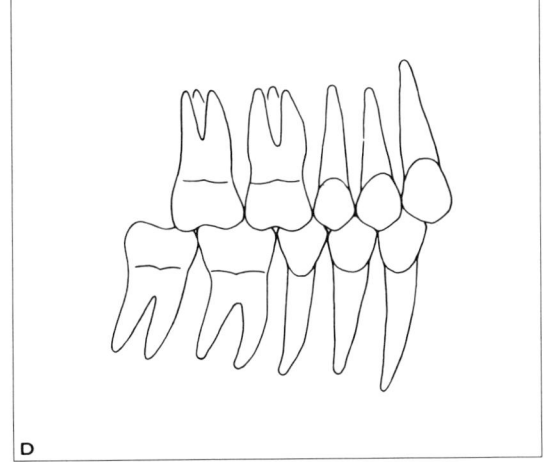

Fig. 10-3 Survey of a Class II/1 malocclusion in the permanent dentition (compare with Fig. 7-1).

A,B Dorsal position of the mandibular dental arch in relation to the maxillary one, abnormally large overjet, and a normal transverse relation between opposing posterior teeth. Normally shaped mandibular dental arch, and a relatively too narrow and tapering maxillary one.

C Increased overbite without vertical support of the mandibular incisors by the lingual surfaces of the maxillary incisors. The incisal edges of the mandibular incisors touch the palate in habitual occlusion.

D In a full Class II relation, as described here, all the mandibular posterior teeth occlude one premolar crown width too far dorsally with the maxillary ones. Nevertheless, the area of intercuspation and the size of the opposing surfaces do not deviate essentially from the Class I situation, except for the last mandibular molar.

Development in Class II/1 Malocclusions

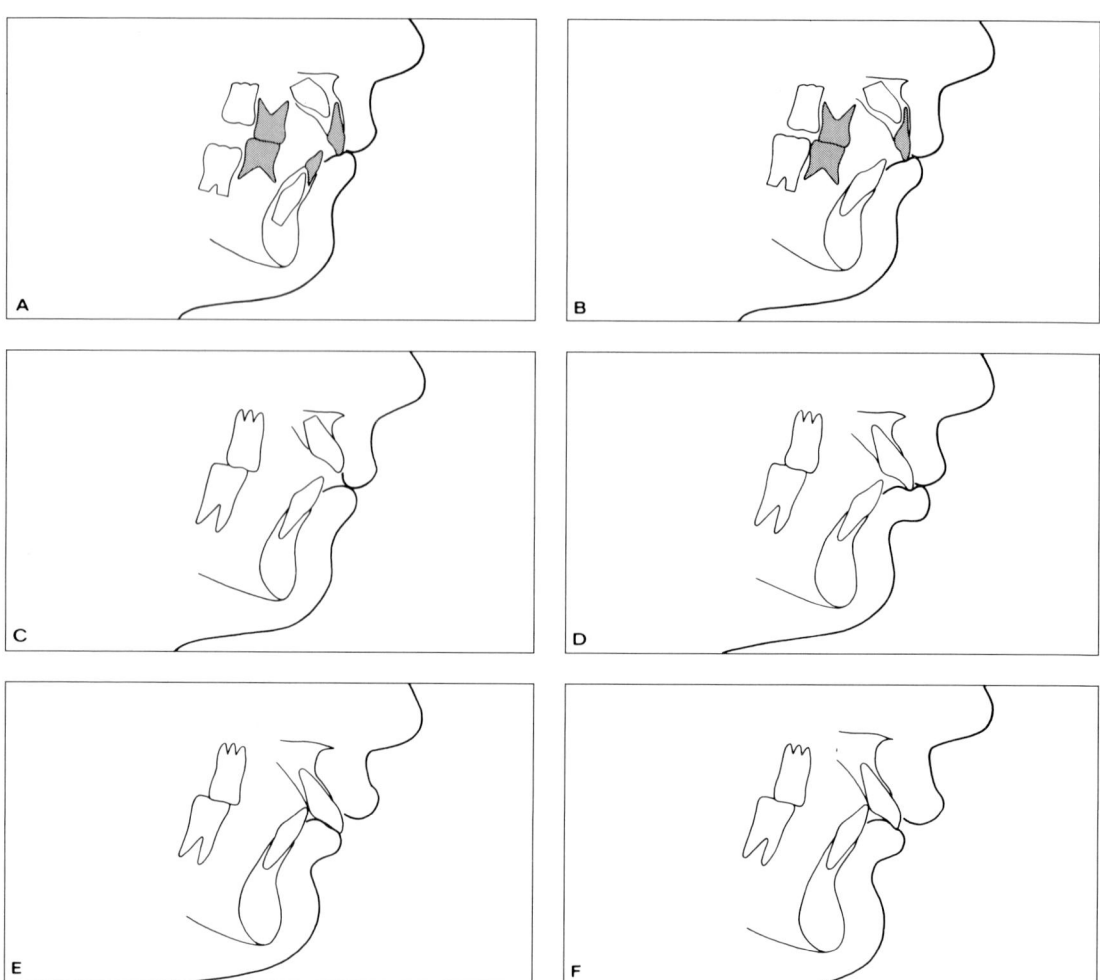

Figure 10-4

Fig. 10-4 Survey of the changes in the incisor and the molar region from the complete deciduous dentition to the adult situation in a Class II/1 malocclusion. The drawings depict cross sections through the right molars, the right central incisors and surrounding bony structures, and the profile (compare with Fig. 4-3).

A   In the complete deciduous dentition, the maxillary deciduous incisors are slightly more labially inclined than normal. An increased overjet exists. Usually, the deciduous incisors do not overerupt until vertically supported contact in occlusion is attained. The terminal plane of the deciduous dentition exhibits a distal step. The lower lip is more dorsally located in relation to the upper lip than is the case in a Class I situation. The anteroposterior position of the lips is determined primarily by that of the two incisor segments.

B   The mandibular first permanent molar has attained the occlusal plane and the mandibular central permanent incisor erupts normally. The maxillary deciduous incisor is vertically in contact with the lower lip.

C   The maxillary first permanent molar has emerged and made contact with its antagonist in a distal occlusal relation of one premolar crown width. Both teeth have large opposing surfaces and intercuspation has been established. The mandibular central permanent incisor erupts further, the maxillary one erupts in a labial direction according to its initial orientation within the jaw.

D   Vertically the mandibular permanent incisor is not supported yet. Its eruption will continue until vertical contact in habitual occlusion is attained. Depending on the local conditions, the central permanent incisor will continue to erupt in its original labial direction or will change in inclination. With thumb sucking—not uncommon in Class II/1 malocclusions—the labial inclination of the maxillary incisors may increase. The lower lip vertically supports the incisal edge of the maxillary incisor.

E   In habitual occlusion, the mandibular incisor touches the palate. In a less severe Class II/1 malocclusion and an associated smaller overjet, the mandibular central incisor will attain contact with the lingual surface of the crown of the maxillary one. The larger the anteroposterior deviation, the more cervically the contact between the opposing incisors will be located at the maxillary incisor crown. In a full Class II molar occlusion, dentally supported incisor contact may exist close to the gingiva palatally to the maxillary incisor. However, under those conditions, contact between the mandibular incisors and the palate (as drawn here) is more usual.

As eruption continues, the maxillary central incisors may become situated in front of the lower lip, as is frequently seen in cases of thumb sucking. Subsequently, the lower lip will further protrude the maxillary incisors and retrude the mandibular ones. An increase of the overjet and secondarily an increase of the overbite will be the result. (However, the latter is usually prevented in cases of thumb sucking, as the thumb then acts as an eruption-inhibiting agent.)

F   In the adult situation, comparatively more lip material is present than during the intertransitional and the second transitional period. The soft tissues continue to increase after the permanent dentition—with the exception of the third molars—has erupted completely. This increase in soft tissue material accounts for the secondary covering of protruding maxillary incisors by the lips often seen during maturation in adolescence.

Development in Class II/1 Malocclusions

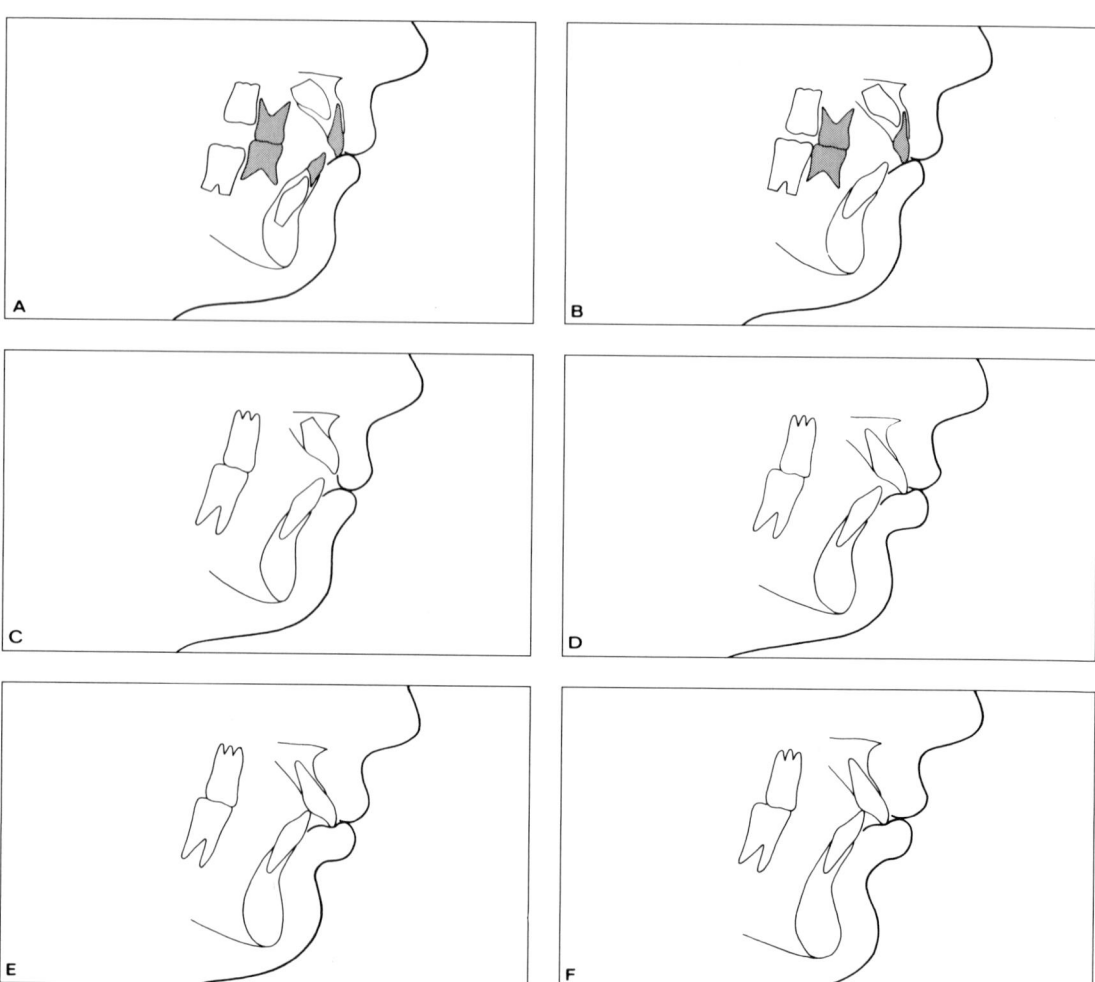

Fig. 10-5 Development, corresponding to that illustrated in Figure 10-4, with the difference that the lower lip does not arrive behind the maxillary incisors. Whether this situation or the one illustrated in Figure 10-4 will be attained depends on a multitude of local factors not discussed here.[102]

of the dentition of a Class II/1 malocclusion as well as in that of a Class I situation. In a Class II/1 malocclusion, with a normally shaped mandibular dental arch and a solid and good transverse intercuspation the maxillary dental arch accordingly will be more narrow than in a Class I situation. The usually narrow and tapering maxillary dental arch in adult Class II/1 malocclusions is not a primary symptom of this malocclusion, but secondarily a derivative of the deviating anteroposterior relation between the two dental arches.

A comparable phenomenon presents itself in the vertical relation of the incisors. Upon emergence, the permanent incisors continue to erupt beyond the usual level because normally dentally supported vertical contact is not attained due to the relatively dorsal position of the mandibular dental arch in relation to the maxillary one. The incisors will continue to erupt until counter pressure is met when the two dental arches are brought into contact with each other. Not only an enlarged overjet will result, but also the overbite will increase abnormally (Fig. 10-5).

Inherent in the deviating sagittal dental arch relation in Class II/1 malocclusions is the absence of a mesial step in the terminal plane of the deciduous dentitions. Different gradations can exist in the configuration of the terminal plane, as a marked variation is found in the severity of Class II malocclusions as a whole. The drawings presented in this chapter are based on a Class II malocclusion in the permanent dentition of a sagittal deviation between the two dental arches of one premolar crown width. However, this is by no means the standard situation. By far most Class II malocclusions present a condition somewhat between a Class I relation and a Class II relation of one premolar crown width. The shape of the maxillary dental arch and the size of the overjet and the overbite are related to the extent of the anteroposterior deviation between the two dental arches and vary accordingly. A smaller deviation in this respect will be accompanied by more moderate secondary symptoms; a larger deviation by more severe ones.

As has been explained above, the primary characteristic of a Class II/1 malocclusion is the dorsal position of the mandibular dental arch in relation to the maxillary one. The other features of a Class II/1 malocclusion are secondary derivatives of the primary characteristic. The same applies to a large extent to the associated tooth-lip relationship. A mild Class II/1 malocclusion is often accompanied by a physiologically normal lip position; a severe Class II/1 malocclusion by a deviating one with the lower lip behind the maxillary incisor crowns. The severity of the Class II/1 malocclusion determines in part whether an initially present abnormal lip position will continue or change to a physiologically normal one when the facial musculature matures during adolescence.

In the presentation of the development of Class II/1 malocclusions in this chapter, it has been assumed that the malocclusion was present from the beginning and did not improve or aggravate subsequently. However, this is by no means always true. During the course of development, Class II/1 malocclusions may improve or be aggravated. The same applies to Class III malocclusions, the development of which will be discussed in Chapter 12.

Development in Class II/1 Malocclusions

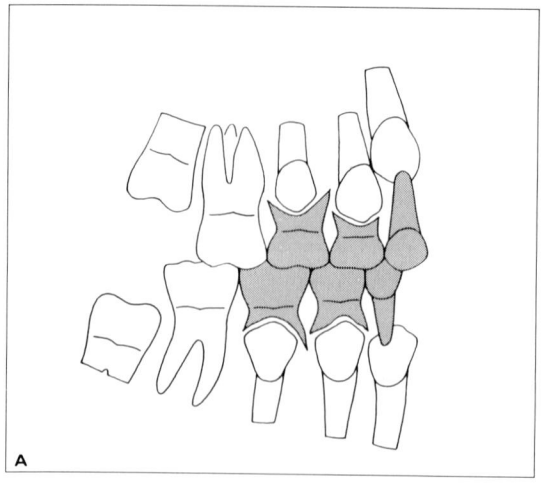

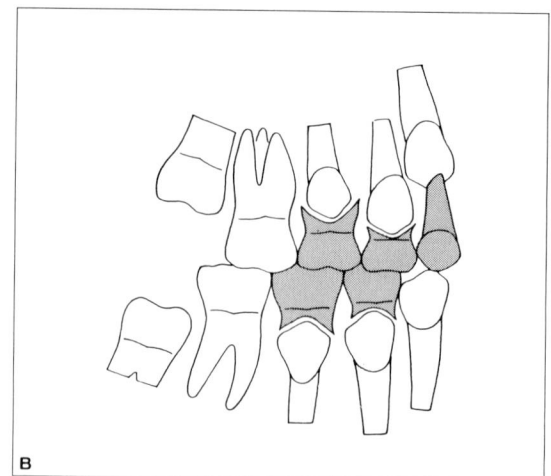

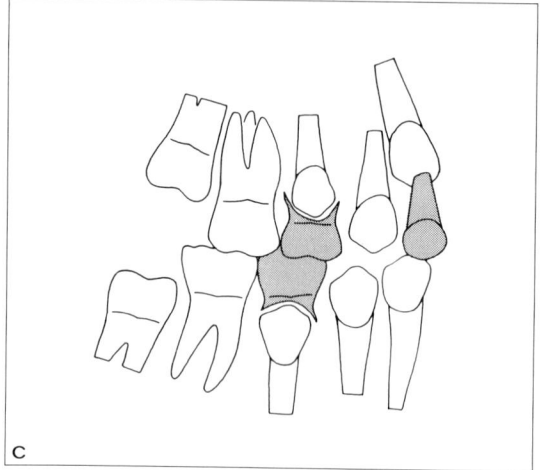

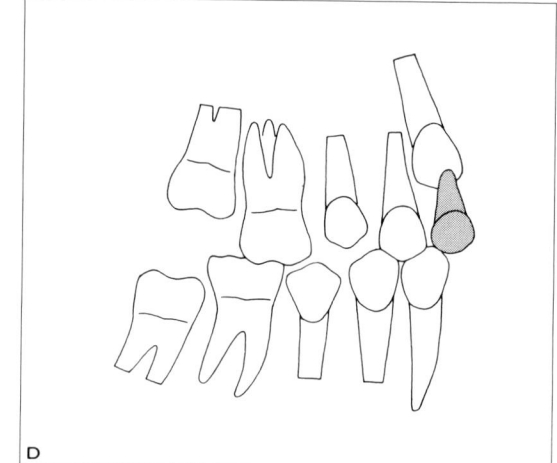

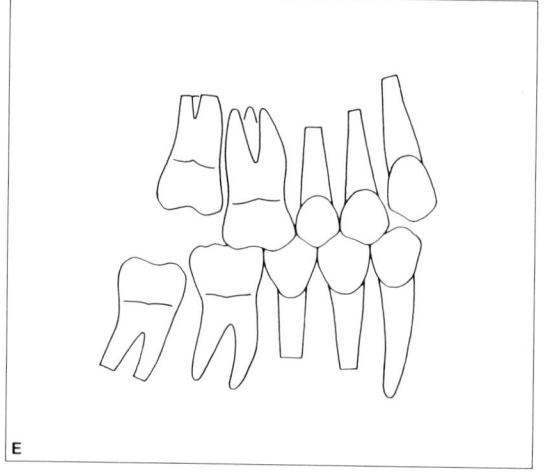

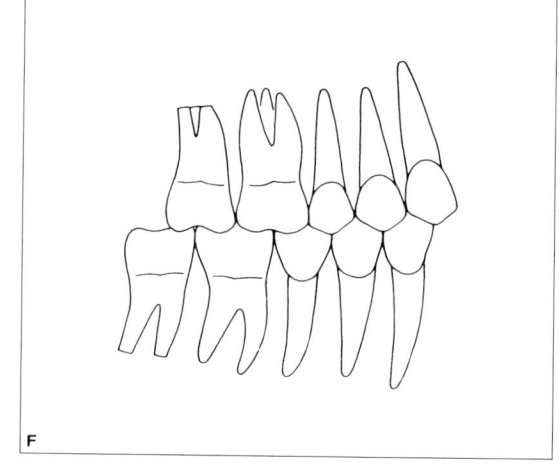

Figure 10-6

Fig. 10-6 Survey of the transition of the posterior teeth and the eruption of the second permanent molars in a Class II/1 malocclusion (compare with Fig. 6-1).

A distinct variation exists in the mesiodistal crown dimensions of corresponding deciduous and permanent posterior teeth, and in the sequence of emergence of the latter (see Chapter 17). The already existing spatial conditions in the dental arch, the size of the extra space derived from the differences in mesiodistal crown dimensions, and the way in which the available space will be filled, determine the shape of the ultimate occlusion. The sequence in transition is of importance, particularly in regard to the consumption of the available space. Occlusion may end up with a less severe deviation, as is illustrated here.

A   The mandibular posterior teeth occlude distally to the maxillary ones. The anteroposterior relation between the second permanent molars still located within the jaws accords.
B   The resorption of the deciduous teeth and the eruption of the successors proceed comparably, as in a normal anteroposterior dental arch relation.
C   After emergence of the first appearing permanent canines and premolars, contact is attained and the previously existing distal relation between opposing deciduous teeth is transferred to their successors.
D   The process continues with the replacement of the other premolars.
E   The maxillary permanent canine attains a mesial relation with the mandibular one instead of a distal relation as is normally the case.
F   Subsequently, the second permanent molars emerge and attain occlusal contact. The distal surface of the mandibular second molar is positioned too far dorsally in relation to the opposing maxillary one and as such extends distally.

The transition of the posterior teeth illustrated here is that of a Class II malocclusion of one premolar crown width (a full Class II occlusion). The ultimate occlusal contact and intercuspation is rather adequate. The opposing cusps of the posterior teeth fit like toothed wheels into each other. In comparison with the normal situation, a shift of one cusp (premolar crown width) exists. In cases with a less severe Class II relation, the opposing posterior teeth occlude in a relation somewhere between the one illustrated here and the normal one (Fig. 6-1). Depending on the severity of the sagittal deviation, the occlusion will be more like a Class I or a Class II situation. In the situation just between the two, the opposing posterior teeth are atop each other in the "end-to-end" relation. Most of the Class II malocclusions are of the end-to-end relation type or nearly so. A full Class II situation as presented here is a truly severe malocclusion and as such does not occur very frequently.

Chapter 11

The Development of the Dentition in Class II/2 Malocclusions

The Class II/2 malocclusion is characterized by a Class II occlusion of the posterior teeth, a distinct retroinclination of two or more maxillary incisors, and a retrusion of the mandibular incisors. However, the most important characteristic of the Class II/2 malocclusion is the high position of the lip line in the median plane (stomion) in relation to the maxillary incisors. Normally the lower and the upper lip contact at a level of one to three millimeters superiorly to the incisal edges of the maxillary centrals. In Class II/2 malocclusions, the lip line is more superiorly located in the median plane and often at the level of the cervical region of the maxillary centrals.
The Class II/2 malocclusion deviates clearly from the Class II/1, not only in its appearance, but also in its development. Futhermore, the dental characteristics of the Class II/2 malocclusion appear in a relatively late phase of the development. Soon after emergence of the maxillary permanent incisors, it becomes obvious in Class II/1 malocclusions that these teeth will protrude too much and that the adequate lip closure may be jeopardized. In Class II/2 malocclusions, the lip closure does not incur a risk.
In Class II/2 malocclusions, three types (A, B, and C) can be distinguished based on differences in the spatial conditions in the maxillary dental arch. In this discussion it is assumed that only in the development of Type A no deviations are originally present in both dental arches.
A Class II/2 malocclusion initially develops as a Class II/1. In the deciduous dentition and in the first transitional period, the normally shaped and sized mandibular dental arch is situated too much dorsally in relation to the maxillary one. The transverse relation between opposing posterior teeth is the same in Class II/2 as in Class II/1 malocclusions. The most important difference in the early developmental stages between the two malocclusions indicated above is formed by the superior location of the lip line. In Class II/2 malocclusions, stomion is often situated at the junction of the

Development in Class II/2 Malocclusions

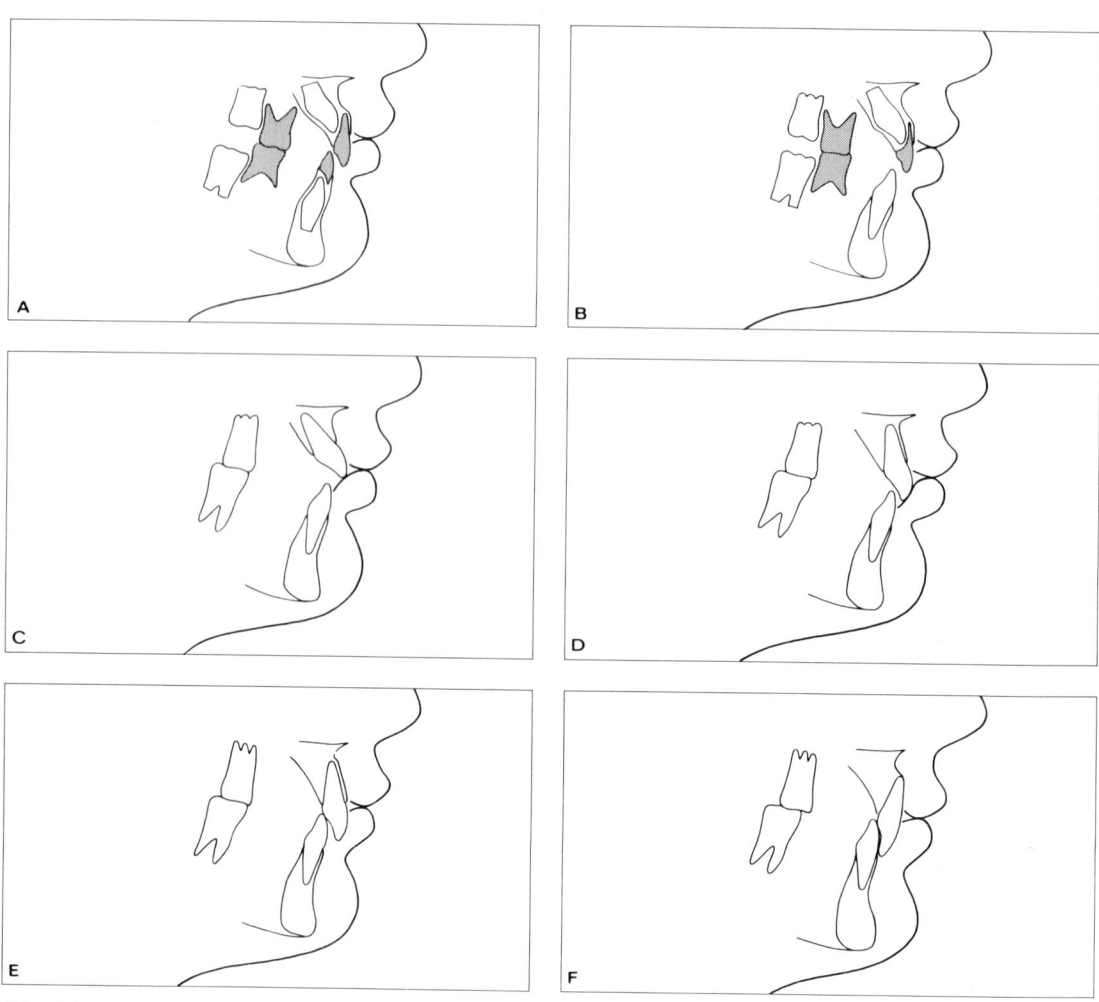

Fig. 11-1

maxillary central deciduous incisor crowns and the labial gingival tissue (Figs. 11-1A and B). In Class II/1 malocclusions, stomion is usually located near the incisal edge of the maxillary central deciduous incisors (Fig. 10-4). In Class II/2 the lower lip covers the labial surfaces of the maxillary deciduous incisors. These teeth are more vertically oriented in the jaw than in a Class II/1 malocclusion. They are also, although

Fig. 11-1 Survey of the changes in the incisor and molar regions in a Class II/2 malocclusion, from the complete deciduous dentition to the adult situation. The drawings are composed of cross sections through the right molars, the right central incisors and surrounding bony structures, and the profile (compare with Figs. 4-3 and 10-4).

A   In the complete deciduous dentition, the maxillary deciduous incisors are slightly less labially inclined than normal. The overjet is somewhat enlarged. Both features differ from the picture in the Class II/1 malocclusion, in which the deciduous incisors are usually somewhat abnormally inclined labially and the overjet is considerably larger than normal. In the Class II/2 malocclusion, the lips are often rather voluminous and the lip line in the median plane (stomion) is situated at the level of the cervical border of the maxillary central deciduous incisors.

B   The mandibular permanent incisor has emerged normally; the maxillary one continues to erupt within the jaw. Prior to emergence, the position of the latter may be normal or slightly more upright. The high lip line relation to the maxillary deciduous incisors is maintained.

C   The maxillary central permanent incisor has emerged according to its previous orientation within the jaw. In accordance with the superior lip line position, the upper lip has only limited effect on the inclination and further eruption of the maxillary centrals. In this stage of development, the lower lip may lead to a limited lingual tipping of the mandibular incisors.

D   The mandibular and maxillary central permanent incisors erupt further. The maxillary central gradually becomes more affected by the lower lip. With continuing eruption of the maxillary central, the size of the contacting area between its crown and the lower lip increases leading to a further lingual tipping of that tooth.

E   Because of the Class II relation between the two dental arches, no sagittal or vertical contact existed between the mandibular and maxillary incisors prior to this stage. The eruption of the incisors has continued until vertical contact has been attained. As a result, the mandibular as well as the maxillary incisors have overerupted. The inclination of the palatally tipped maxillary incisor is unfavorable for supporting the mandibular incisor vertically. Upon the attainment of sagittal contact between the mandibular and maxillary central incisors, the pressure of the lower lip will also lead to a lingual tipping of the mandibular teeth as the force is transmitted through the maxillary teeth, which continue to tip palatally.

F   In the adult situation, the maxillary central incisor is tipped severely palatally and its labial surface is completely covered by the lower lip. The lower lip does not, or only in a very limited way, support the maxillary central incisor vertically. The maxillary incisors may contact the gingiva labially to the mandibular ones. In a comparable way, the maxillary central incisor received little or no support vertically from the mandibular incisors, which in turn usually contact the palatal mucosa.

slightly, more vertically oriented than in patients with normal development of the dentition (Fig. 4-3).

Upon emergence, two or more maxillary permanent incisors tip palatally under influence of the abnormal lip position and the forces exerted by the lower lip on the maxillary incisors (Fig. 11-1;[31,36,37,47,60,75]). Some changes occur in the

Development in Class II/2 Malocclusions

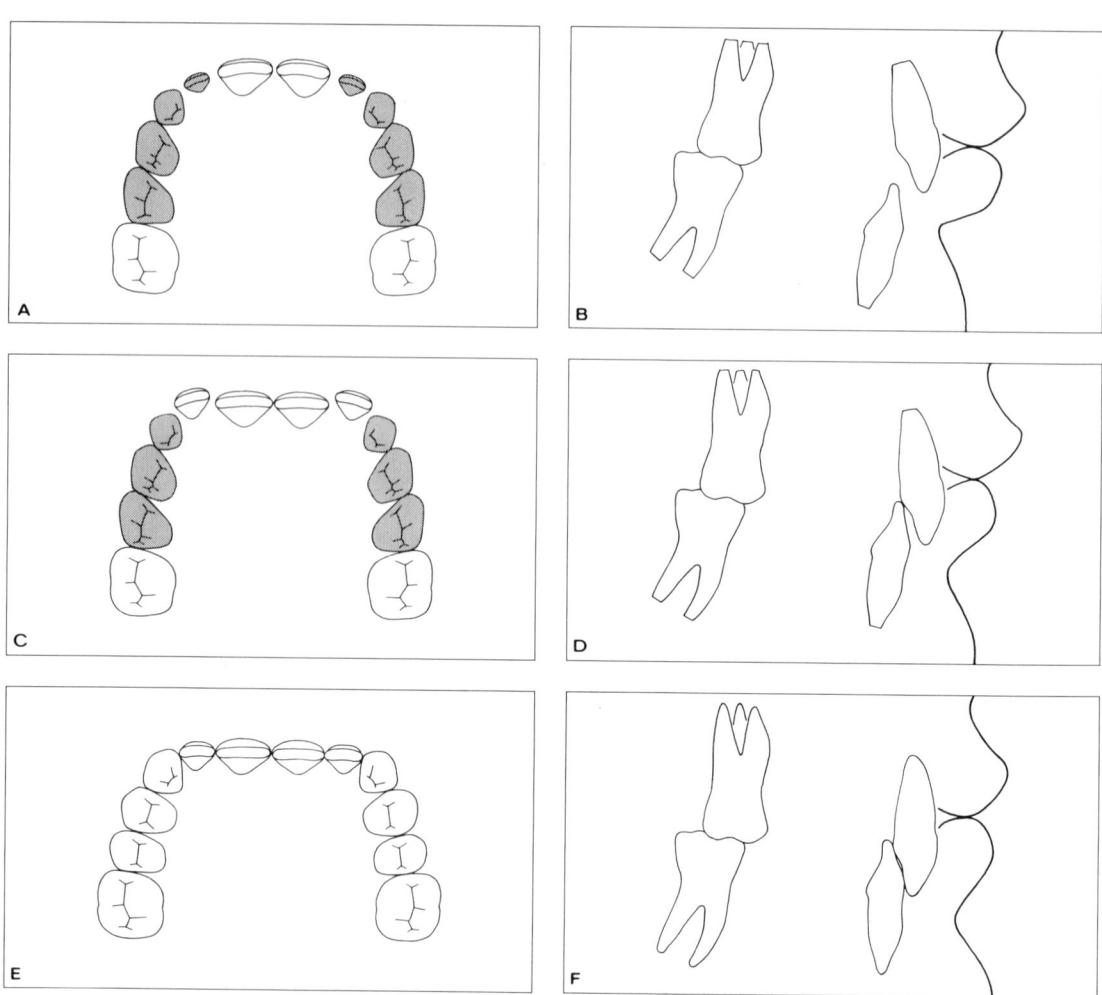

Figure 11-2

maxillary dental arch, resulting again in alterations in the mandibular arch. By the palatal tipping of the maxillary centrals, the contacting mandibular incisors also will be moved lingually. The change in arch form from a half round shape to a more rectangular one is not limited to the maxillary dental arch. The man-

Fig. 11-2 Survey of the changes in the maxillary dental arch in the incisor region in a developing Class II/2 malocclusion with more than sufficient space in its anterior segment (Type A). In this figure and in the two following, the deciduous teeth have been shaded in the occlusal views.

A,B The maxillary permanent central incisors have emerged and erupted to the level of the occlusal plane. They are located harmoniously in the dental arch. The maxillary deciduous laterals are not yet shed. More than sufficient space is available for their successors. The lower lip covers more than half of the labial surface of the maxillary incisors. Some lingual tipping of these teeth has already taken place. Normally, the maxillary central permanent incisors emerge more labially in the dental arch than where their predecessors were located (see Figs. 4-3 and 8-2A and C). Through the lingual tipping already caused by the lower lip, the maxillary central permanent incisors form a continuous arch with the deciduous lateral incisors and canines.

C,D The maxillary lateral permanent incisors have emerged according to their original orientation within the jaw; they erupt more labially than where their predecessors were located. More than sufficient space in the dental arch is available for the laterals even after the maxillary centrals have been tipped more palatally. Under these conditions, the labial surfaces of the further erupting lateral incisors may also become covered by the lower lip. Concomitantly, the laterals will tip palatally gradually and will undergo a process comparable to that begun by the maxillary central incisors a year earlier, one that is not yet completed by far. In the meantime, the mandibular incisors have erupted further. After contact has been attained between the mandibular and maxillary incisors, the former are tipped lingually by the lower lip through forces transmitted by the latter.

E,F In the adult situation, the maxillary laterals are tipped palatally in the same manner and to a comparable degree as the centrals. Seen from the occlusal side, the incisal edges of the four maxillary incisors more or less form a straight line. Adequate space was left for the permanent canines to emerge within the dental arch. Through the palatal tipping of the four maxillary incisors, the shape of the dental arch has been changed to a more rectangular form. The mandibular and maxillary incisors are oriented approximately perpendicularly to the occlusal plane and do not, or only slightly, support each other in vertical direction.

dibular one undergoes a comparable change in shape. In cases with an excess of space in the maxillary dental arch (Type A), the four maxillary permanent incisors can tip palatally without occurence of crowding (Fig. 11-2). A comparable picture applies to the mandibular dental arch.

Development in Class II/2 Malocclusions

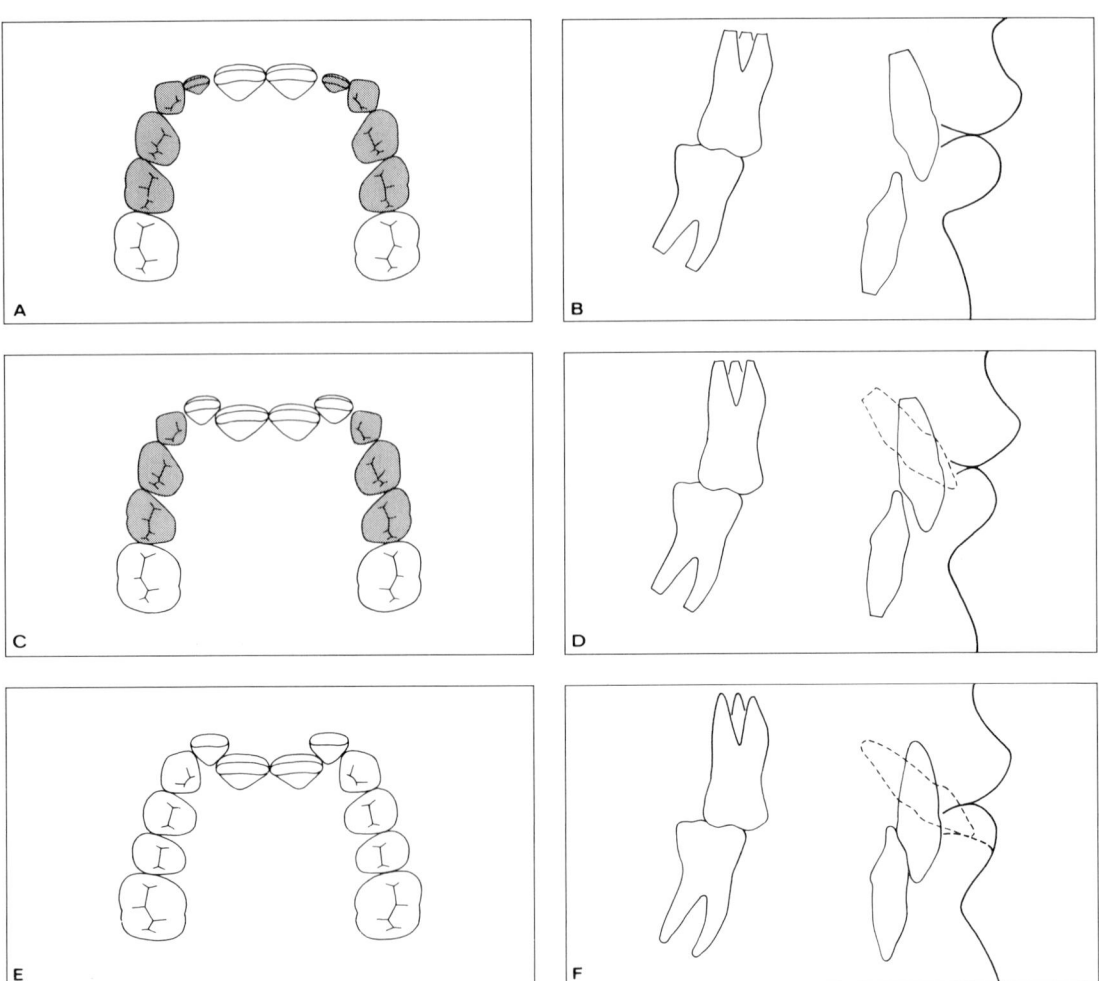

Figure 11-3

In combination with the high lip line position and the lingual tipping of the incisors, a certain excess of external soft tissue material often seems to be present in the anterior region in Class II/2 malocclusions. The lips attain a more dorsal position and a "dished-in" appearance may develop. The lower lip may be rather voluminous and, moreover, often exerts a larger force on the adjacent teeth than in Class I or Class II/1 situations.[79]

Development in Class II/2 Malocclusions

Fig. 11-3 Survey of the changes in the maxillary dental arch in the incisor region in a developing Class II/2 malocclusion with crowding in its anterior segment (Type B). The maxillary lateral permanent incisors are indicated with a dotted line in D and F.

A,B The central permanent incisors have emerged and subsequently have been tipped palatally. They form a harmonious continuous arch together with the deciduous lateral incisors and canines. Normally, the maxillary central permanent incisors should have been situated more labially. Too little space is available in the dental arch for the not yet emerged maxillary permanent laterals. Vertical contact has not yet been attained in the incisor region. The mandibular permanent incisors and maxillary central ones erupt further. Concomitantly, the lower lip gradually covers a larger surface of the maxillary central incisors, which continue to tip palatally.

C,D The already limited space for the maxillary lateral permanent incisors in the dental arch has been reduced even more by the continuing palatal tipping of the central ones. In the eruption after emergence, the laterals evade labially. The lower lip becomes positioned lingually to the maxillary lateral incisor crowns. This is more likely to be the case if the lip line at the corners of the mouth is more inferiorly situated than in the median plane, as is usually characteristic in the development of Class II/2 malocclusions of Type B. The labial inclination of the maxillary laterals is aggravated by the palatal position of the lower lip behind them. The maxillary centrals and the mandibular incisors continue to erupt and will attain contact.

E,F In the adult situation, the maxillary central incisors and the four mandibular incisors are about perpendicularly oriented to the occlusal plane. Often, vertical contact exists between the incisal edges and the gingiva, labially to the mandibular incisors and palatally to the maxillary ones. The maxillary laterals are distinctly labially inclined and rest on the lower lip, which covers the labial surfaces of the centrals completely. The combination of the inferior position of the lower lip in the region of the laterals with the superior position of the centrals forms an essential feature in the development of the process described above. Crowding in the maxillary dental arch is usually associated with crowding in the mandibular one. An already existing crowding in the mandibular dental arch will worsen considerably from the lingual tipping of the mandibular incisors.

In Type B, the available space in the maxillary dental arch is limited. The maxillary central permanent incisors will move palatally gradually after emergence. However, in crowded conditions, this movement will decrease the already limited space for the lateral permanent incisors further. Consequently, the laterals cannot move palatally and will evade labially (Fig. 11-3). The lower lip will become positioned inferiorly to the maxillary lateral incisors and as such will contribute to the increase of their labial inclination.

Development in Class II/2 Malocclusions

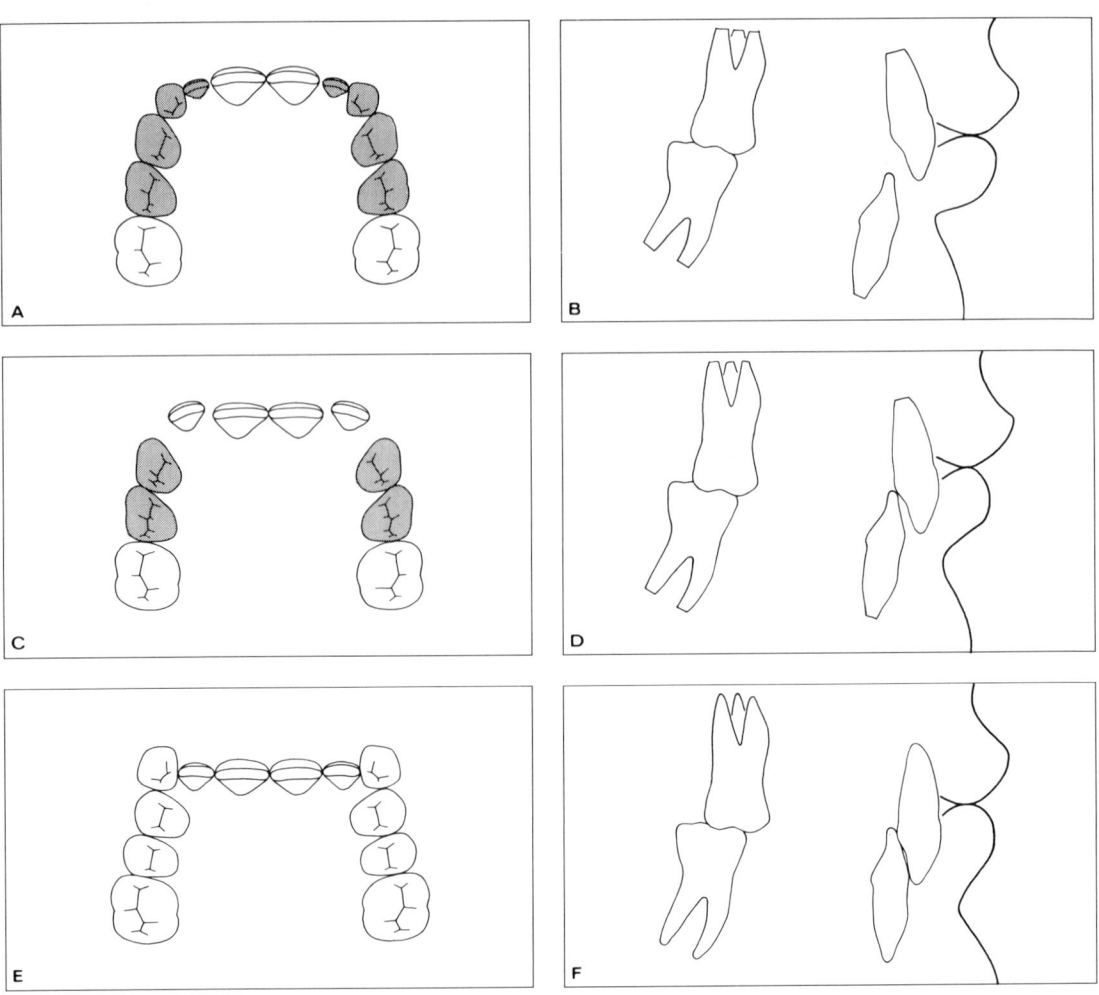

Figure 11-4

Type C develops in instances with a marked shortage of available space in the maxillary dental arch. Prior to emergence, the erupting maxillary lateral permanent incisors may not only lead to resorption and shedding of their predecessors, but of the adjacent deciduous canines as well. The latter will be lost prematurely with the effect that extra space becomes available for the palatal

Fig. 11-4 Survey of changes in the maxillary dental arch and in the incisor region in a developing Class II/2 malocclusion with premature loss of the maxillary deciduous canines. Their roots were resorbed in association with the eruption of the lateral permanent incisors (Type C).

A,B The maxillary permanent centrals have emerged and more than half of their labial crown surfaces is covered by the lower lip. The maxillary centrals have been tipped palatally by the forces exerted by the lower lip. Considerable lack of space exists in the maxillary dental arch prior to the emergence of the permanent laterals. The available space is reduced even more by the continuing palatal tipping of the maxillary centrals during further eruption and the increase of the surfaces covered by the lower lip.

C,D An occurrence associated with emergence of the lateral permanent incisors is that not only the roots of their predecessors but also those of the adjacent deciduous canines have been resorbed. By the shedding of the deciduous canines in addition to the laterals, sufficient space becomes available for the permanent laterals to emerge and erupt within the dental arch without meeting obstacles. Initially, the permanent laterals erupt in the usual labial direction, conforming to their orientation within the jaw prior to emergence. However, their crowns gradually become covered by the lower lip, as happened previously to the centrals. Consequently, the laterals tip palatally. This movement can be executed because extra space has become available by the premature loss of the deciduous canines.

E,F The space remaining for the permanent canines to emerge and attain a proper position in the dental arch is markedly deficient. The canines have emerged in buccal direction. Their mesial surfaces are visible and their cusp tips extend in a disturbing way. In addition, the canine crowns are positioned more labially than those of the four maxillary incisors that have been tipped palatally and whose incisal edges form more or less a straight line. At completion of the development of the dentition, vertical contact has been attained between the incisal edges and the gingiva in the mandible and the maxilla. Initial crowding in the maxillary dental arch usually is associated with crowding in the mandibular one. The lingual tipping of the mandibular incisors will increase the already present crowding in the mandibular dental arch. The process described here is more likely to occur in subjects in whom transverse configuration of the lip line is such that there is less chance of the lower lip becoming positioned lingually to one or both maxillary lateral incisors (compare with Fig. 11-3).

tipping of the maxillary lateral permanent incisors. The lower lip will not only tip the maxillary centrals, but also the laterals palatally. The space destined for the not yet emerged maxillary permanent canines in the dental arch becomes more and more reduced. Later, they will emerge buccally and attain positions outside the dental arch (Fig. 11-4).

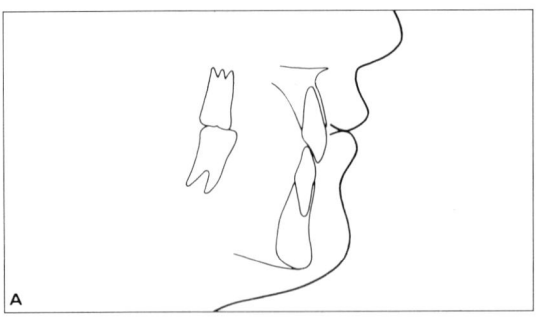 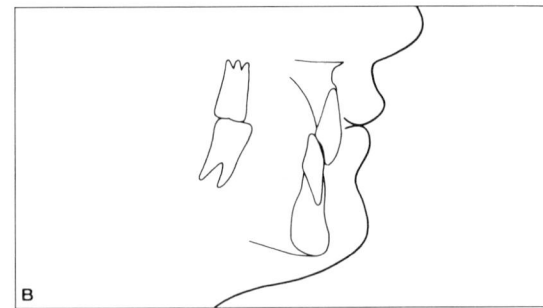

Fig. 11-5 Survey of the changes in the inclination of the mandibular and maxillary incisors during the last phases in the development of the dentition of Class I malocclusion with Class II/2 symptoms.

A The preceding phases in the development of the dentition are comparable to those shown in Figures 11-1A to D, with the major difference being that the occlusion in the molar region is not a Class II but a Class I. The superiorly positioned lip line has had the same effect on the maxillary incisors as has been described before. In a normal sagittal dental arch relation, contact between the mandibular and maxillary permanent incisors will be attained shortly after emergence. Initially, some dental support is present in vertical direction. However, this support is insufficient to inhibit the eruption movements. Moreover, the maxillary incisors are not supported vertically by the lower lip in the normal way.

B Concomitantly with the increase in size of the surfaces of the maxillary central incisors covered by the lower lip, these teeth continue to tip palatally. The force of the lower lip is transmitted through the maxillary incisors to the contacting mandibular ones. As a result, the latter also tip more lingually, and to a larger degree than is the case in a Class II/2 malocclusion, as the tipping starts earlier. In Class II/2 malocclusions, sagittal contact between maxillary and mandibular incisors is attained at a later stage, as the overjet is larger initially.

The phenomenon of a high lip line position is not exclusively reserved for Class II occlusions. It can also be encountered in a Class I relation between the two dental arches. In those circumstances, development is comparable with that of Class II/2 malocclusions, with two main differences. The sagittal occlusion of the molars, and later also of the premolars, will be normal; the mandibular incisors will be tipped more lingually (Fig. 11-5). The cases described here are indicated as Class I malocclusions with Class II/2 symptoms.

Conformable to the approach followed in the discussion of the development of the Class II/1 malocclusions in the preceding chapter, the development of the Class II/2 malocclusion has also been concentrated on the severe abnormality associated with a full Class II occlusion. However, less severe forms of Class II/2 malocclusions also occur. Likewise, a certain scale exists not only in regard to the severity of the Class II relation between the two dental arches, but also the degree of lingual inclination of the maxillary and mandibular incisors. The variation in lingual inclination depends mainly on the degree of overlap of the maxillary incisors by the lower lip. If the lower lip covers more than one-third of the labial surface of the maxillary central incisor crowns, the lingual tipping of these teeth as described here is likely to take place.

Chapter 12

The Development of the Dentition in Class III Malocclusions

A Class III malocclusion is characterized by a ventral position of the mandibular dental arch in relation to the maxillary one. In comparison with the normal situation, the mandibular posterior teeth occlude too much mesially with the maxillary ones. In the incisor region, a reversed overjet exists with the incisal edges of the mandibular incisors ventrally to those of the maxillary ones. As has been explained before, the Angle Classification leaves undecided whether the primary factor that caused the malocclusion is located in the mandible, the maxilla, or in a combination of both. This etiological neutrality holds equally true for Class III as well as Class II malocclusions.
Theoretically, it could be stated that in Class III malocclusions as well as in Class II/1 malocclusions, the shape of the mandibular dental arch is basically normal as seen occlusally. However, this is not the case. In Class II/1 malocclusions, a normal though enlarged anteroposterior relation between the maxillary and mandibular incisors exists, resulting secondarily in an increased overjet and overbite. Viewed occlusally, the shape of the mandibular dental arch is not or only slightly influenced by the occlusion. This is not the case in the Class III malocclusions, as reversed anteroposterior relation of the incisors is accompanied by significantly deviating occlusal contacts. In the development of a Class III, the maxillary and mandibular incisors can become displaced reciprocally. These changes are not limited to the maxillary dental arch, but also involve alterations in the location of several teeth in the mandibular arch. Diastemata may develop in the mandible, particularly in cases with no shortage of space for the mandibular teeth.
As in the discussion of the development of the dentition in Class II/1 malocclusions, the discussion of Class III malocclusions starts with the situation in the deciduous dentition (Fig. 12-1), followed by the intertransitional period (Fig. 12-2), and the permanent dentition (Fig. 12-3). Subsequently, the eruption of the first permanent molars and the transition of the incisors is described (Fig. 12-4). Finally, the transition of the posterior teeth is treated (Fig. 12-5).

Development in Class III Malocclusions

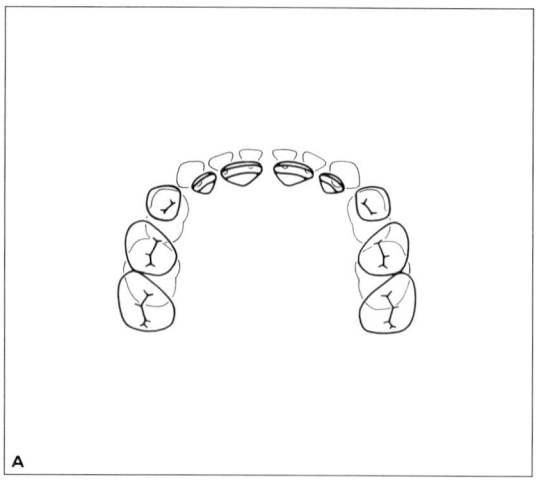
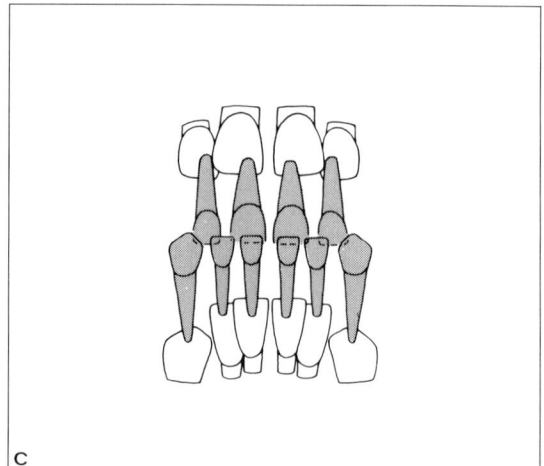
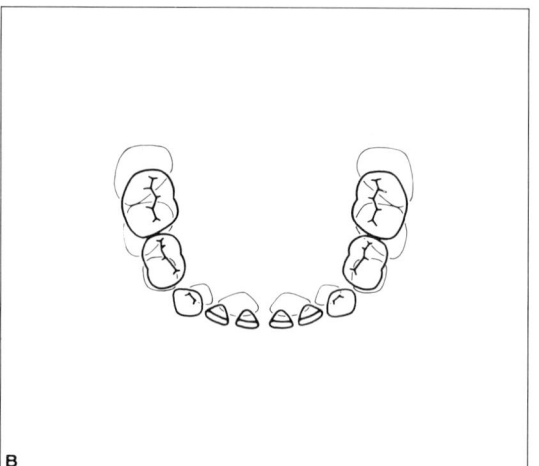
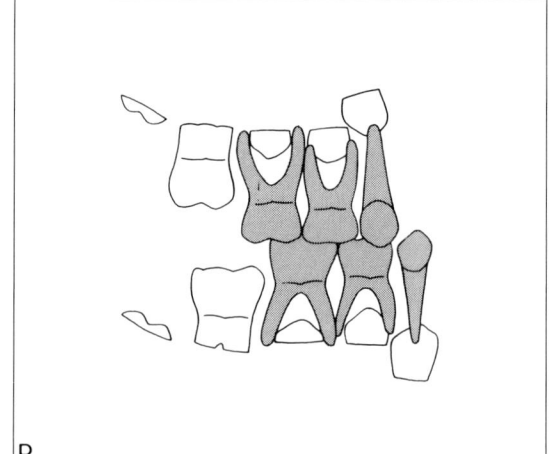

Fig. 12-1 Survey of a Class III malocclusion in the complete deciduous dentition (compare with Fig. 3-1).

A,B The mandibular dental arch is too far ventral in relation to the maxillary one. A good transverse relation exists between the mandibular and maxillary deciduous molars. The opposing four mandibular incisors and canines are situated in a reversed overjet (anterior cross bite).

C The mandibular incisors and canines are situated ventrally to the maxillary ones. A limited overbite is present.

D The mandibular deciduous molars occlude too far mesially to the maxillary ones. The terminal plane of the deciduous dentition shows an abnormally large mesial step.

Development in Class III Malocclusions

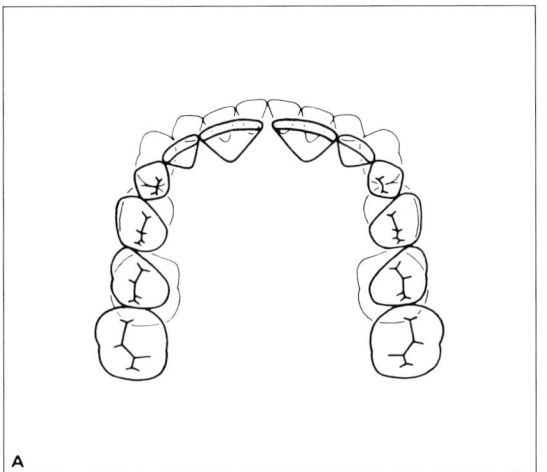
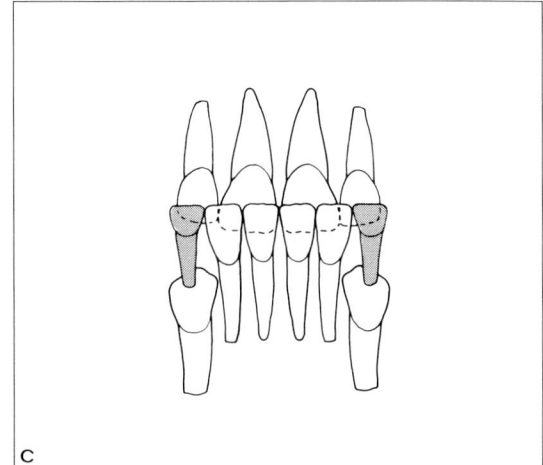
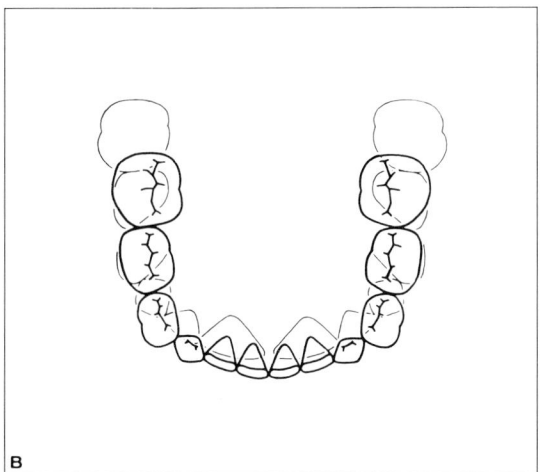
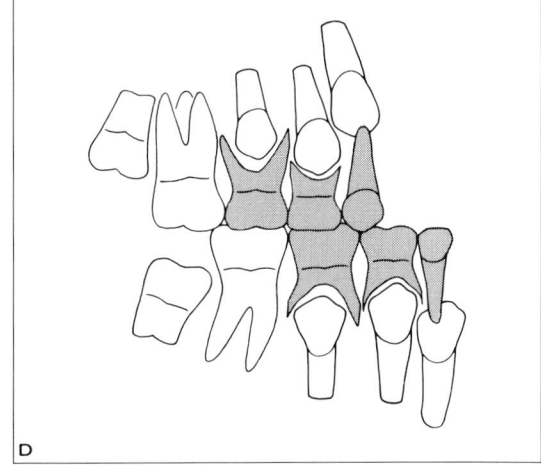

Fig. 12-2 Survey of a Class III malocclusion in the intertransitional period. In comparison with the illustration in Figure 12-1 of the deciduous dentition, the malocclusion has aggravated considerably (see also Fig. 5-1).

A,B *Ventral position of the mandibular dental arch in relation to the maxillary one. Reversed overjet in the incisor-canine region. The individual position of the teeth is in accordance with the deviation in contacts and the crossing over of the occlusion in the canine region.*
C *The mandibular and maxillary incisors have erupted further. The incisal edges of the maxillary incisors contact the lingual surfaces of the mandibular incisors.*
D *The mandibular first permanent molar occludes too far mesially to the maxillary one. The contact surface between them is small.*

Development in Class III Malocclusions

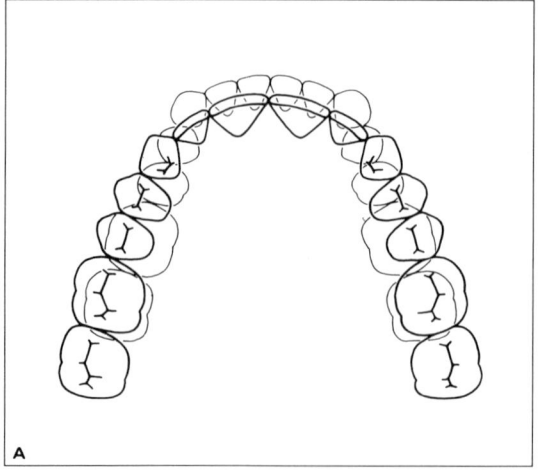
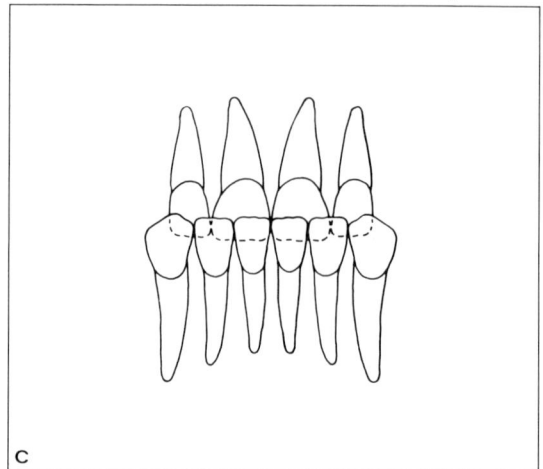
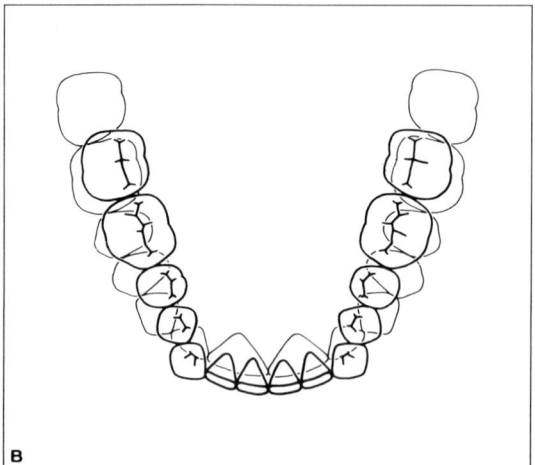
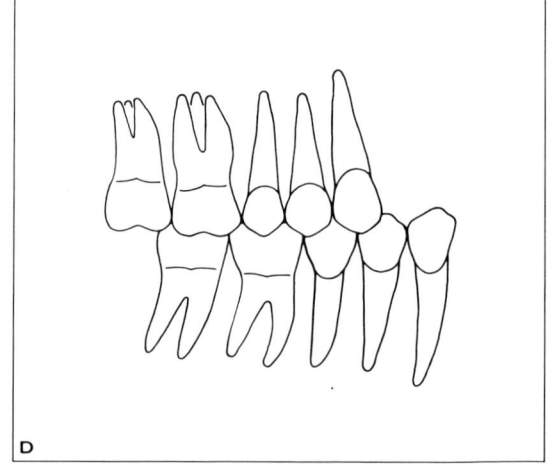

Fig. 12-3 Survey of Class III malocclusion in the permanent dentition (compare with Fig. 7-1).

A,B Ventral position of the mandibular dental arch in relation to the maxillary one; reversed overjet in the anterior region. The position of the individual teeth is adapted to the deviations in occlusal relations.
C Also the mandibular permanent canines are positioned labially to the maxillary lateral incisors.
D All posterior teeth occlude too much mesially by one premolar crown width.

Class III malocclusions can be more severe than the one illustrated here. The sagittal deviation between the two dental arches can be larger than one premolar crown width. Under these conditions, the posterior teeth usually occlude transversally in a reversed relation (posterior cross bite). This deviation in transverse relation of the posterior teeth may also occur in less severe malocclusions than the one illustrated here.

The relation between the lower and upper lip in Class III malocclusions clearly deviates from the normal picture. The lower lip is more ventrally positioned than the upper lip. In combination with the often dominating chin, the reversed lip relation leads to the typical facial appearance and profile that are characteristic of the Class III malocclusion (Fig. 12-4).

The reversed overjet of the incisors is associated with a lip-teeth relation that differs markedly from the normal situation. Consequently, the ventral and vertical support of the incisors by the lips differs accordingly. More related information is provided in Figure 12-4. The presentation of the development of the Class III malocclusions is based on a deviation in the anteroposterior dental arch relation of one premolar crown width in the adult situation. In Class III malocclusions, many degrees of severity also are encountered, although less evenly distributed than in Class II malocclusions. In the latter, the size of the anteroposterior deviation between the two dental arches varies more according to a continuous distribution; in the former the distribution is partially discontinuous in character. The discontinuous nature is caused by the fact that the anterior cross bite forms a distinct reversal point between the Class I situation and the Class III dental arch relation.

The transverse relation between the opposing posterior teeth can be abnormal from the very beginning when the first deciduous molars attain occlusal contact. The mandibular first deciduous molars may extend buccally over the opposing maxillary ones in both sides of the jaw. This reversed transverse relation may be continued when the occlusion of the second deciduous molars is attained subsequently, and later when the permanent molars are added to the dental arches. Under these circumstances the mandibular dental arch is broader than the maxillary one. Not only are the incisors situated in a reversed position, but the posterior teeth contact each other in such a way that the mandibular teeth are abnormally buccally positioned in relation to the maxillary ones.

The anteroposterior relation between the two dental arches is mainly determined by the way contact is reached when the mandible is closed under normal conditions with the mandibular condyles properly located in the temporal fossae. It may happen that in a normal closing movement of the mandible, contact is made initially between the two dental arches before maximal occlusion is attained. The initial contact interferes with the continuation of the normal closing movement. In the succeeding movement, the mandible will slide ventrally or laterally or in a combined direction. Subsequently, maximal vertical contact will be reached in a position deviating from the normal path of closure. This deviation in closure movement, which can be diagnosed as a sliding after an initial contact has been reached is called a "forced bite." Forced bites are frequently encountered in deviating jaw relations between a Class I and a Class III dental arch relation of one premolar crown width (anterior forced bite). In these circumstances, the initial contact is usually situated in the incisor region.

The individual location of teeth in both dental arches depends mainly on the occlusal contact. Large variations exist in this respect; these will not be explored here. The anterior forced bite is treated in Chapter 14, as is the Class III subdivision.

Development in Class III Malocclusions

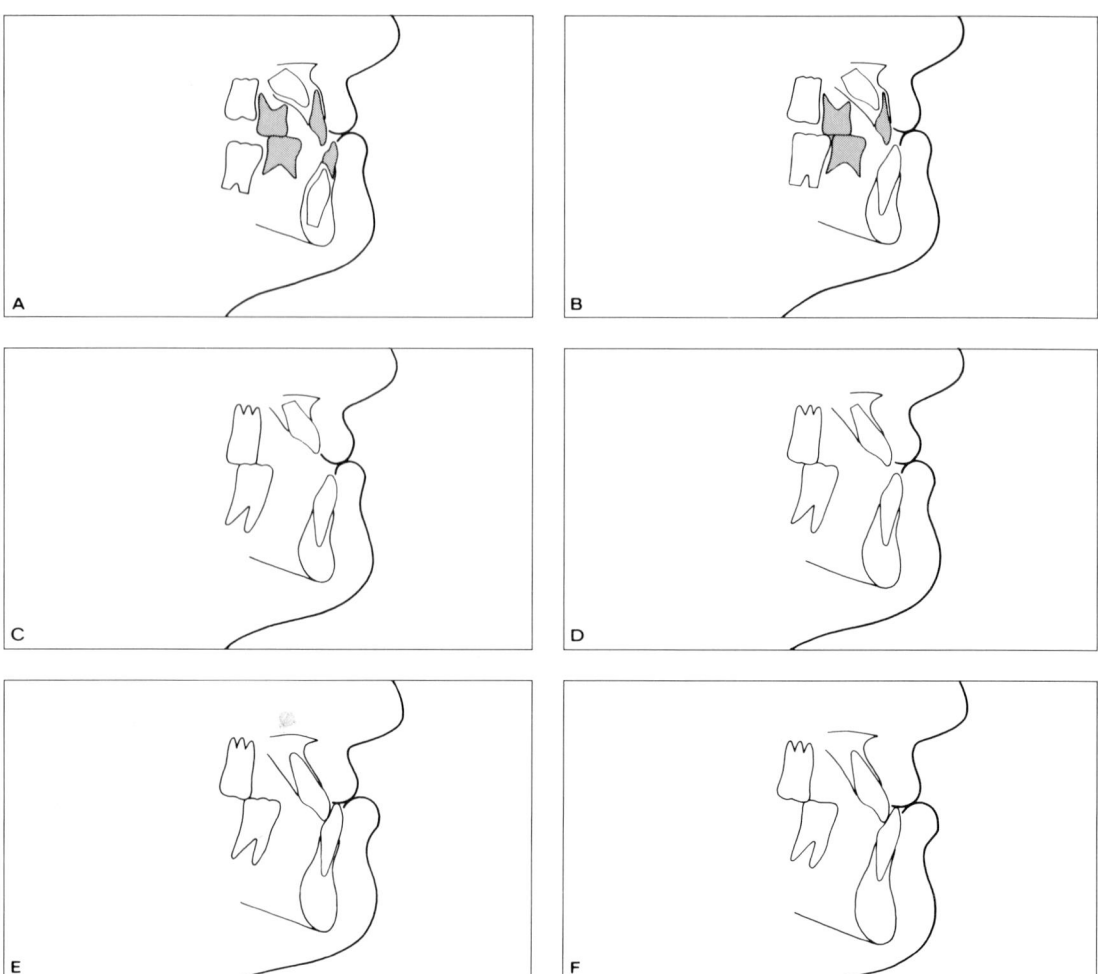

Figure 12-4

Fig. 12-4 Survey of changes in the incisor and molar region from the complete deciduous dentition to the adult situation in a progressively aggravating Class III malocclusion. The drawings have been composed from cross sections through the right molars, the right central incisors and surrounding bony structures, and the profile (compare with Fig. 4-3).

A In the complete deciduous dentition, the maxillary deciduous incisors are slightly more labially and the mandibular ones slightly more lingually inclined than normal. A reversed overjet (anterior cross bite) exists. Contact between the incisors often is not present. The permanent incisors are located within the jaws in a normal position and inclination. The terminal plane of the deciduous dentition has an abnormally large mesial step.
The anterior surface of the lower lip is located more ventrally than that of the upper lip.

B The mandibular first permanent molar has attained the occlusal plane. The mandibular central permanent incisor erupts normally. The lower lip does not contact the maxillary central deciduous incisors.

C The maxillary first permanent molar has emerged and attained contact with its antagonist in an abnormal sagittal relation. The mandibular central incisor erupts further. The maxillary one has emerged in accordance with its initial orientation within the jaw.

D The maxillary central incisor does not contact the lower lip in the continuation of its eruption movement. Hence, the lower lip does not affect, or only slightly, the inclination of the erupting maxillary incisor. Neither the maxillary incisor nor the mandibular one are supported vertically.

E The mandibular and maxillary central incisors have erupted further and attained contact. The labioincisal edge of the maxillary incisor touches the lingual surface of the mandibular incisors. The size of the reversed overjet as well as the amount of vertical overlap (overbite) are determined in part by the sagittal relation between the two dental arches and in part by the prevailing local conditions in the dental arches. The tongue also plays an essential role in this respect. In comparison with the normal situation, the maxillary incisors are tipped more labially and the mandibular ones more lingually in Class III malocclusions. Generally, the larger the sagittal deviation between the two dental arches, the more the inclination of the incisors is affected. The maxillary incisor is supported vertically by the contact with the mandibular incisors. Reciprocally, the mandibular incisor is supported by the maxillary one. Furthermore, the former is additionally supported vertically by the upper lip. The degree of vertical support and the associated amount of overbite can vary considerably.

F In the maturation to the adult situation, the typical features of the Class III malocclusion profile usually are intensified. By an increase in soft tissue material, the lower lip usually becomes more protruded. The late growth of the face results in a larger dominance of the chin in ventral direction.

In these six drawings, the Class III malocclusion worsened during the process of growth and development, as is often actually the case.

Development in Class III Malocclusions

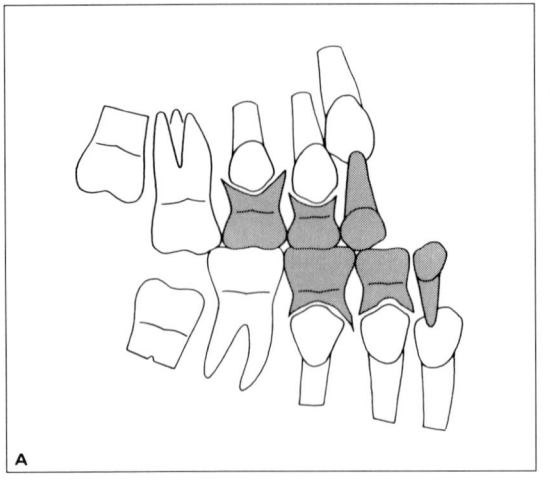
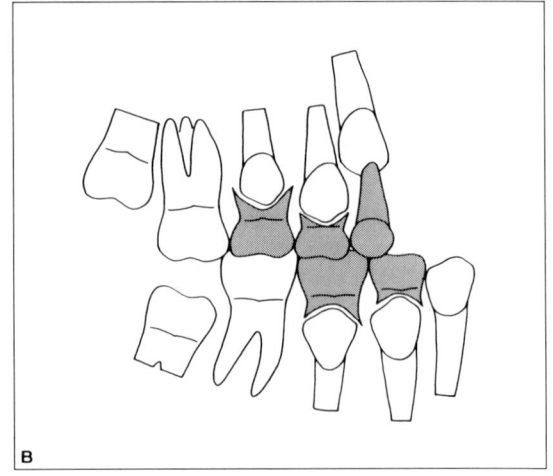
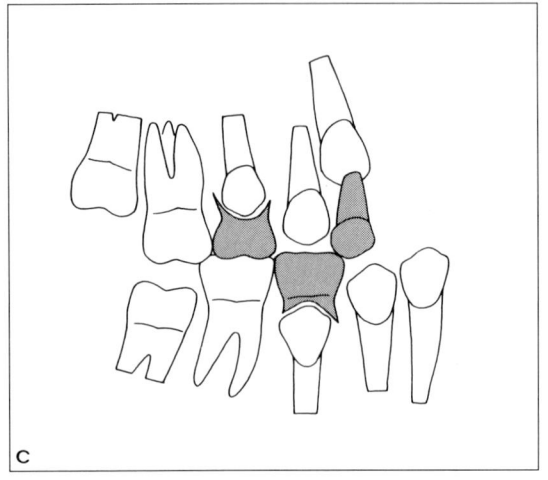
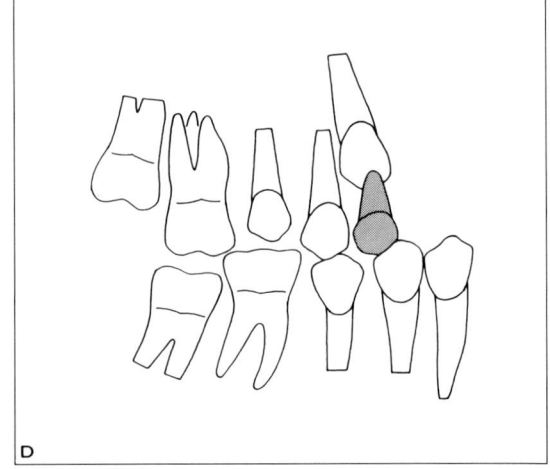
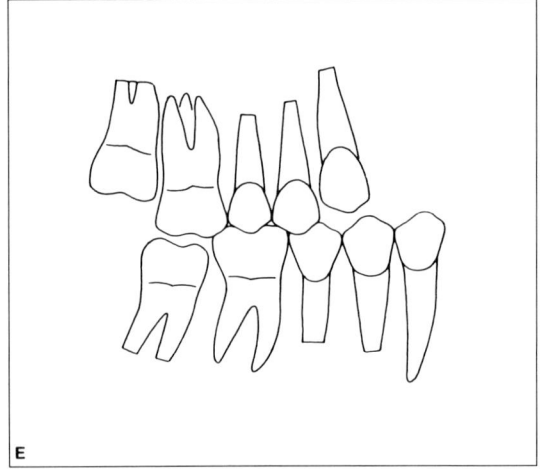
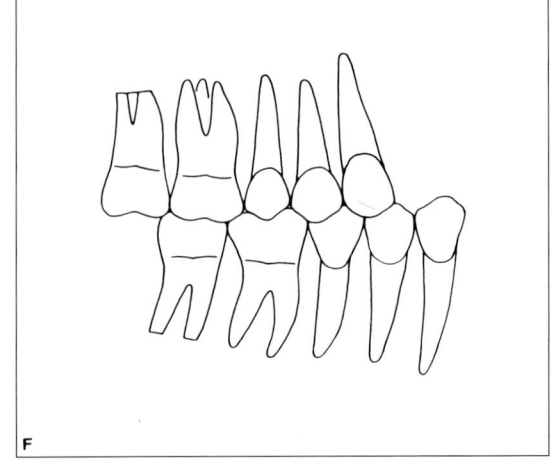

Figure 12-5

Fig. 12-5 Survey of the transition of the posterior teeth and eruption of the second permanent molars in a Class III malocclusion that did not worsen during the second transitional period (compare with Fig. 6-1).

A The mandibular posterior teeth occlude abnormally mesially to the maxillary ones. The anteroposterior position of the not yet emerged second permanent molars corresponds.
B The resorption of the deciduous teeth and the eruption of their successors proceed in a manner comparable to the one in a normal sagittal dental arch relation.
C Upon emergence of the permanent canines and premolars first to appear, contact is attained in the abnormal sagittal relation. The deviating mesial occlusion between the mandibular and maxillary posterior teeth is continued and confirmed.
D The same process takes place upon emergence of the remaining premolars.
E The maxillary permanent canine will occlude distally to the mandibular first premolar.
F Subsequently, the second permanent molars emerge and attain occlusion. As is the case for the first molars, the second ones contact each other only over a small surface. To the contrary, a large contact area exists between the mandibular second permanent molar and the maxillary first one.

The transition of the posterior teeth illustrated here is that of a Class III malocclusion of a complete premolar crown width. Under these circumstances, a rather good occlusal contact and intercuspation can develop. Frequently, the posterior teeth arrive in a transverse abnormal relation and the mandibular molars and premolars extend buccally to the maxillary ones in a posterior cross bite.

Class III malocclusions may aggravate progressively during growth and development. They may end up with a larger sagittal deviation between the two dental arches than one premolar crown width. The variation in Class III malocclusions in the range between a Class I and a Class III occlusion of one premolar crown width is restricted by the reversing point associated with the anterior cross bite. As such, the variation is smaller than that encountered in Class II malocclusions for the corresponding range size. As has been explained in Chapter 10, all stages between a Class I and a full Class II occlusion can be encountered in Class II malocclusions because no phenomenon comparable to a reversed overjet interrupts the continuum within the range.

Development in Class III Malocclusions

A Class III malocclusion may worsen during the course of development. The anteroposterior relation between the two dental arches can worsen in time because of an abnormally large ventral growth of the mandible, a retardation in ventral development of the maxilla, or a combination of both. The sagittal deviation between the two dental arches in Class III malocclusions can exceed one premolar crown width.

Coincidentally with the worsening of the deviating sagittal relation between the two dental arches, an initially normal sagittal relation of the anterior teeth and a transverse relation of the posterior teeth can become abnormal. In a progressively developing Class III, the replacement of the deciduous incisors by the permanent ones may be associated with a changeover of the overjet. An initial normal overjet can become a reversed one during transition. A comparable phenomenon may happen in the posterior region. Deciduous molars that were situated in a normal transverse relation may become replaced by premolars that occlude in a transverse reversed way.

In the adult dentition the Class III malocclusion is characterized by an abnormal labial inclination of the maxillary incisors and an abnormal lingual inclination of the mandibular incisors. The larger the sagittal deviation between the two dental arches, the larger these deviations in inclination. In a way, the deviation in sagittal relation between the two dental arches is compensated by the adaptation in labial inclination. The tongue and the lower lip probably play an essential role in the attainment of the labial inclination of the maxillary and mandibular incisors, which is typical for a Class III adult malocclusion.

Chapter 13

The Development of the Dentition in Open Bites

An *open bite* can be defined as a lack of normal vertical contact between opposing teeth over a limited region or, as seldom occurs, over the total dental arch. The concept of open bite also covers the lack of vertical contact between the teeth and the gingiva, if further eruption should have resulted in contact between the teeth and the gingiva. This condition may occur in a severe Class II/1 malocclusion with a large overjet in which the mandibular incisors have not fully erupted. Then the incisal edges of the mandibular incisors do not reach the palate. Some space remains in between.
An open bite is most frequently seen in the anterior region, mainly due to abnormal habits such as thumb or finger sucking. In these cases, the open bite is usually asymmetrically shaped. The position of the teeth and the deformation of the alveolar processes exhibit a configuration that represents more or less an impression, a negative of the thumb or fingers as they were placed in the mouth during sucking (Fig. 13-1).
Moreover, an open bite in the anterior region may also be caused by positioning of the anterior part of the tongue between the incisal edges of the mandibular incisors and the lingual surface of the maxillary incisors during normal, relaxed circumstances. When the tongue is placed between the incisal edges of the mandibular and maxillary incisors, the open bite may be so large that the incisors do not overlap vertically when the posterior teeth are brought into occlusion. In open bite subjects, the tongue is placed between the teeth to obtain an adequate seal of the anterior part of the mouth. Children with anterior open bites caused primarily by abnormal sucking habits also swallow with the tongue positioned in the open bite space to achieve an adequate enclosure. Generally, an open bite caused by a sucking habit will close spontaneously if the abnormal habit is eliminated, unless the abnormal tongue position is maintained.
An open bite can be encountered in all distinguishable types of jaw relations and occlusal conditions. It is frequently associated with a Class II/1 mal-

Development in Open Bites

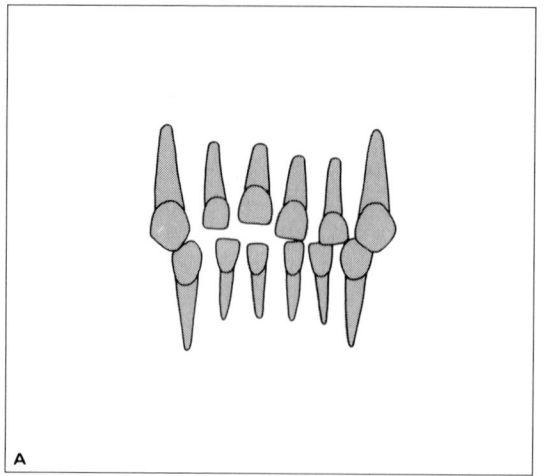
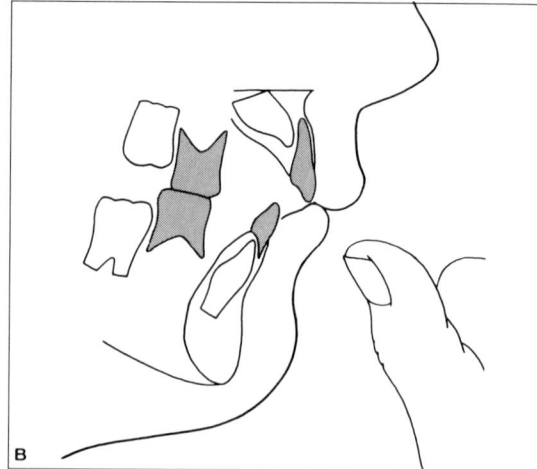
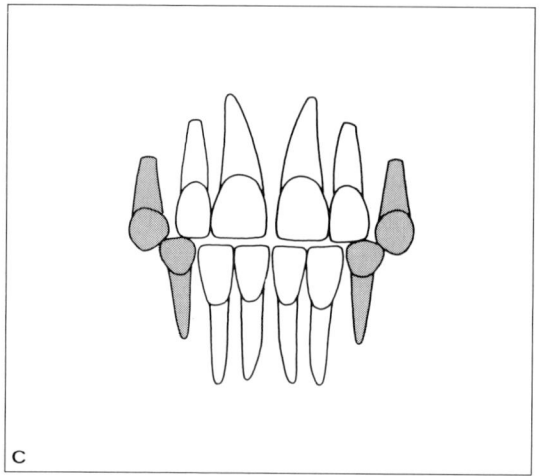
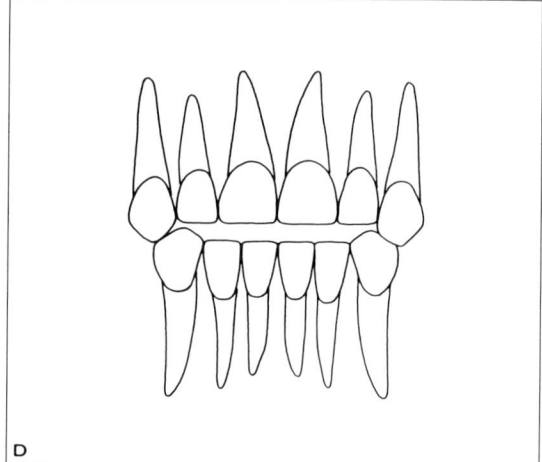

Fig. 13-1 Simplified presentation of anterior open bites.

A,B Asymmetrical open bite caused by thumb or finger sucking. This form of open bite is frequently seen in the deciduous dentition. If the sucking habit is not terminated at an early age, the permanent incisors will attain a comparable open bite position after they have replaced their predecessors.

C,D Open bite due to an abnormal tongue position. This type of open bite is usually symmetrical in shape and can vary in size considerably. Vertical overlap of the opposing incisors may be present or absent.

occlusion. The size of the open bite can vary considerably and may range from a few millimeters to more than one centimeter. A small open bite is occasionally present in a Class II/1 malocclusion with the incisal edges of the mandibular incisors in close proximity to, but not in contact with, the palate. A large open bite can be encountered, for example, in a Class I situation with no vertical overlap of the opposing incisors at all, but a distance of one centimeter between them (Fig. 13-2).

Open bites in the posterior regions are caused by incomplete eruption of the teeth resulting from interpositioning of the tongue. The open bite can be limited to two opposing teeth or involve a larger area (Fig. 13-3). An open bite in the posterior region can be combined with inadequate contact. Then the opposing teeth touch each other, however, in an abnormal and incomplete way. An open bite in the posterior region may be caused by an interpositioning of the tongue between the lingual cusps of the opposing premolars, while their buccal cusps touch with their cusp tips. Usually the pertaining teeth are abnormally related in transverse direction also. The tongue has interfered with attainment of the cone-funnel mechanism.

Anterior open bites are usually present from the beginning of the development of the dentition. They are most frequently seen in the deciduous dentition. When the open bite is caused exclusively by thumb or finger sucking, the open bite usually corrects spontaneously when the abnormal habit is terminated. Also, the protrusion and asymmetrical position of the maxillary incisors usually disappear naturally. These corrections usually take place spontaneously if the abnormal habit is stopped prior to the transition of the incisors.[111] However, in later phases correction may still occur.

Anterior open bites caused exclusively by an abnormal position of the tongue are usually symmetrical in shape, in contrast with the ones caused primarily by an abnormal habit (see Fig. 13-1). When the abnormal position of the tongue dissolves, the open bite will correct spontaneously.

A special form of local open bite is caused by the arrest of eruption of a tooth due to the development of a bony union between the cementum of the tooth and the adjacent bone *(ankylosis)*. This phenomenon is often seen in a mandibular second deciduous molar. Its vertical development remains behind that of the other teeth and contact with the antagonist is lost. Gradually, the distance between its occlusal surface and the occlusal plane increases. The ankylosed tooth becomes submerged. Adjacent teeth also may become ankylosed and a more extensive open bite will develop. Single-tooth ankylosis and combined ankylosis of adjacent teeth not only occur in deciduous teeth, but also in permanent ones (see Fig. 9-6).

Open bites are not always easy to diagnose, particularly in lateral open bite instances. Situations with no maximal occlusal contact of the posterior teeth are suspect in this regard. The same applies to abnormal transverse relations of posterior teeth (Fig. 13-3). A narrow maxillary dental arch with the opposing posterior teeth positioned approximately atop each other in transverse direction (end-to-end) is almost always related to an abnormal tongue position.

Open bites in the posterior regions can be partial or complete. In diagnosing these conditions, the situation on the other side of the dental arches can serve as a valid

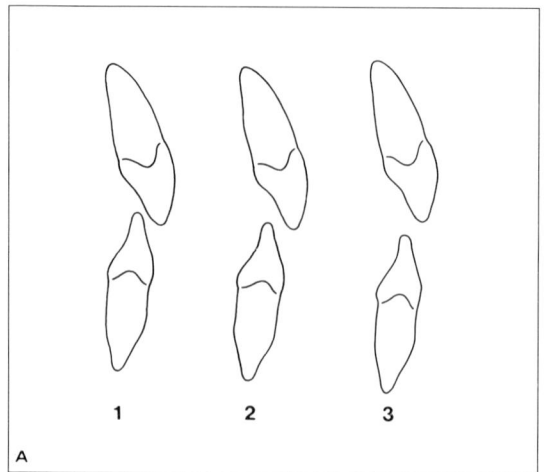
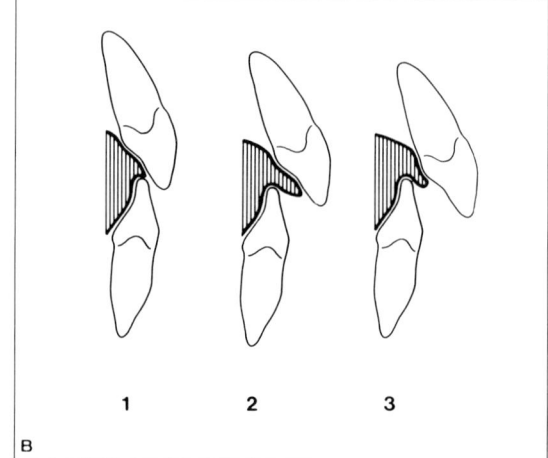

Fig. 13-2 Survey of some variations in anterior open bites in different sagittal relations between the two dental arches.

A   An open bite caused by thumb or finger sucking is usually rather large (A-3). The opening is large enough to accommodate the thumb or fingers comfortably in the mouth without opening the mandible inconveniently far. In an open bite caused by an abnormal tongue position, the size of the opening that is maintained depends on the degree in which the tongue is positioned between the mandibular incisors, the maxillary incisors and the palate. In cases with a limited interpositioning of the tongue, the open bite will be small (A-1). In cases with a rather voluminous tongue, of which quite a large part is positioned between the mandibular incisors and the maxillary ones, a large open bite may result. (A-2).

B   A small open bite in a Class I situation (B-1); a moderate open bite in a Class II malocclusion (B-2); and a moderate open bite in a Class II/1 with a large overjet. Note the variation in the degree of vertical overlap of the opposing incisors.

Development in Open Bites

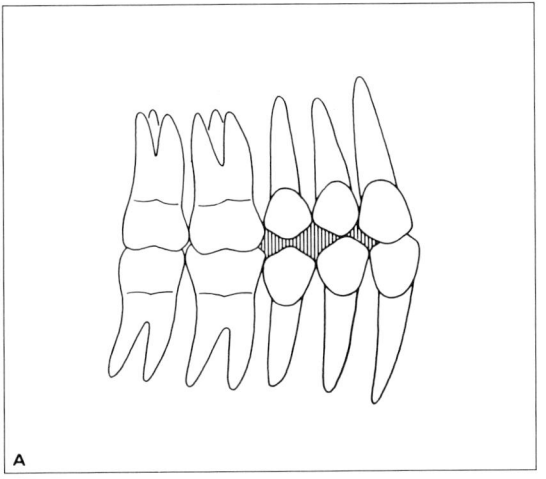
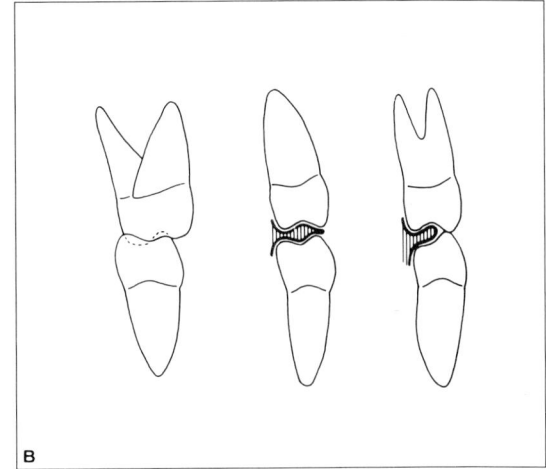
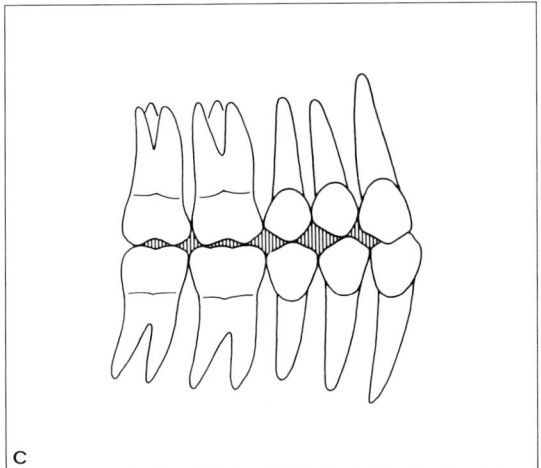
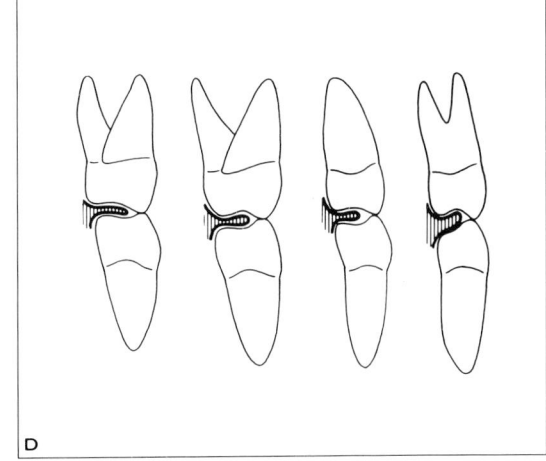

Fig. 13-3 Simplified presentation of open bites in the posterior regions.

A,B Local open bite in the right posterior region with complete absence of contact between the second premolars and inadequate contact between the first premolars. In contrast with the premolars, the first permanent molars intercuspate properly and have been guided in a good transverse relation (B).

C,D Open bite on the right side with inadequate contacts between the opposing mandibular and maxillary teeth. No good transverse relation and intercuspation has been achieved.

guide and as a basis for comparison. An open bite in the posterior region can also be present bilaterally in a partial or complete form. Only the anterior region may have vertical contact. A unilateral open bite may be combined with one in the anterior region. The total open bite is the most extreme form, in which none of the teeth makes normal contact. In diagnosing a total open bite, the absence of a good transversal relation between the posterior teeth and the lack of maximal possible contacts in the posterior and anterior regions are important criteria. A particular problem in the diagnosis of open bites is the unrealistic impression that is obtained when patients are asked to put the teeth into contact. In response to that request, they usually place the tongue inside the dental arches; the teeth are brought into contact and may touch on several points, and the total open bite does not show up as such.

The development of open bites is not further explored for Class II and Class III malocclusions. The various aspects of the open bite explained above can be thought to be superimposed on the development of the dentition in Class II/1 and Class III malocclusions, as has been discussed before.

Finally, it may be noted, that a certain type of open bite is associated with an abnormal growth direction of the mandible, in which the chin moves primarily inferiorly. In these instances, even a maximal eruption of the teeth may not prevent the development of an open bite. This type of open bite has not been incorporated in this discussion.

Chapter 14

Subdivisions (Angle), Forced Bites and Deviations in Transverse Dental Arch Relations

The contents of this chapter are not focused on developmental aspects but more on some consequences of certain deviations in the relationship between the two dental arches.

As has been indicated before, Angle supplemented his classification with subdivisions. In the Class II/1 subdivision (Fig. 14-1), a normal sagittal relation of the posterior teeth is present on one side and a Class II occlusion on the other. A corresponding situation exists in a Class III subdivision, in which a normal sagittal relation of the posterior teeth is present on one side and a Class III occlusion on the other (Fig. 14-2). According to Angle, a situation with a Class II occlusion on one side and a Class III on the other does not ccour.[1]

In a *forced bite,* the normal closing movement of the mandible cannot be continued in the intended direction of movement. The two dental arches make initial contact at one or more points. Subsequently, the mandible glides into a position in which more contact is reached between the mandibular and maxillary teeth.

Forced bites can be distinguished in lateral and anterior ones and in a combination of both. In a lateral forced bite, first the posterior teeth usually attain contact when a normal closing movement is performed. Subsequently, the mandible glides laterally. A lateral forced bite is generally associated with a maxillary dental arch too narrow in comparison with the mandibular one. When maximal occlusal contact is established, a reversed transverse relation is present on one side. Also, the midpoints of the mandibular and maxillary dental arches do not match (Fig. 14-3).

In anterior forced bites, the initial contact is usually attained in the incisor-canine region. Subsequently, the mandible glides ventrally. In general, the result is an anterior cross bite *(progenic forced bite*—Fig. 14-4). However, an anterior forced bite can also exist in a Class II/1 malocclusion with crowding in the maxillary anterior region. When both dental arches are brought into maximal contact, the Class II occlusion appears less severe or is even fully masked, and a Class I

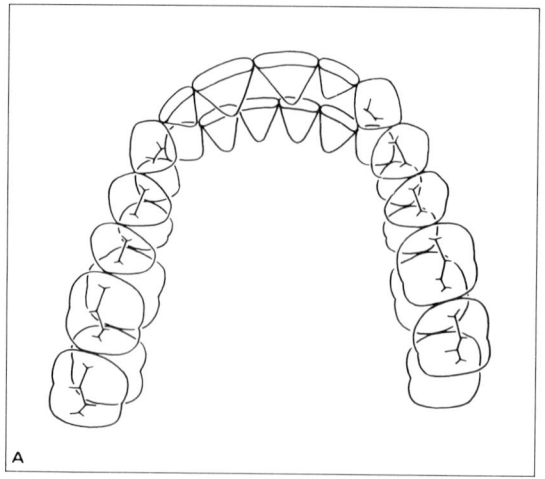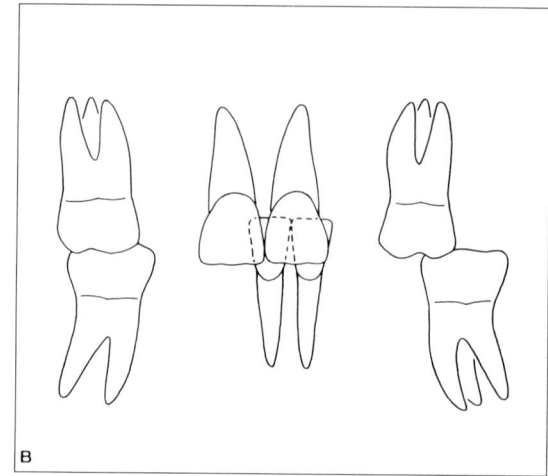

Fig. 14-1 Schematic presentation of a Class II/1 subdivision.

A   The posterior teeth show a normal transverse relation. In sagittal direction, a Class I molar occlusion exists on the right side, a Class II on the left.
B   The overjet and overbite are too large; the midpoints of the two dental arches do not match.

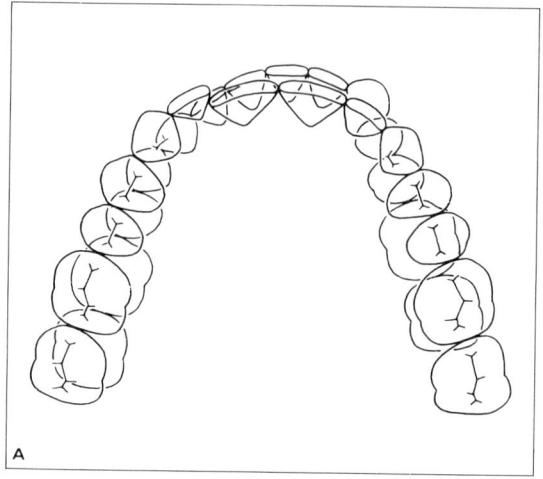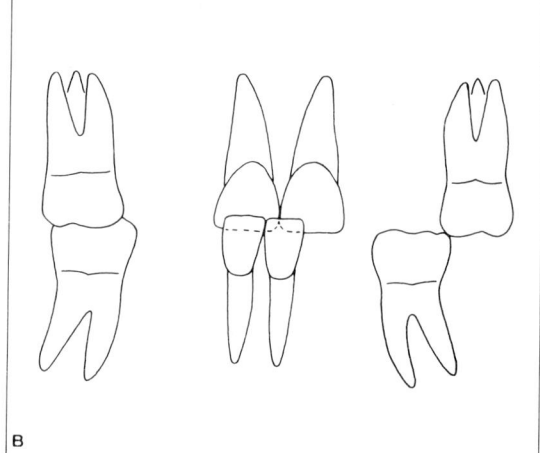

Fig. 14-2 Schematic presentation of a Class III subdivision.

A   A Class I molar occlusion on the right side, a Class III on the left.
B   The midpoints of the two dental arches do not match; an anterior cross bite exists for the majority of the incisors and the left canines.

Subdivisions, Forced Bites and Transverse Deviations

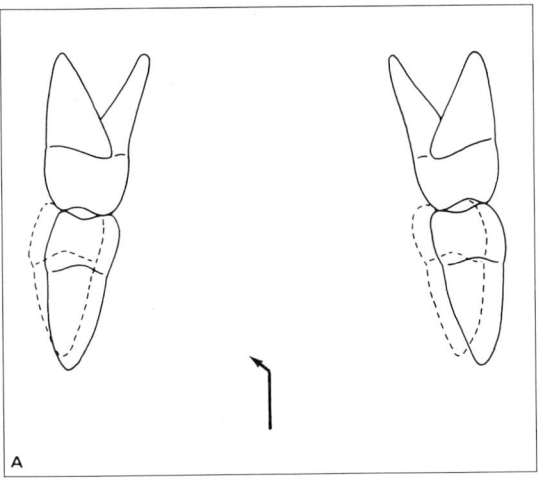 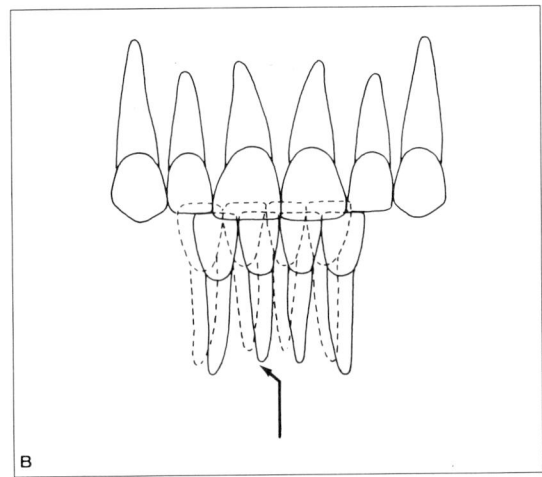

Fig. 14-3 Schematic presentation of an example of a lateral forced bite. The mandibular teeth are drawn with continuing lines in the initial contact situation and with dotted lines in the habitual occlusion. The path of closure is indicated by an arrow.

A   In the normal closing movement, initial contact is reached in the posterior regions between the cusp tips. Subsequently, the mandible glides to the right side, and more contact between the two dental arches is attained on both sides. In habitual occlusion, an abnormal transverse relation exists unilaterally in the form of a posterior cross bite on the right side.

B   The midpoints of the two dental arches deviate accordingly.

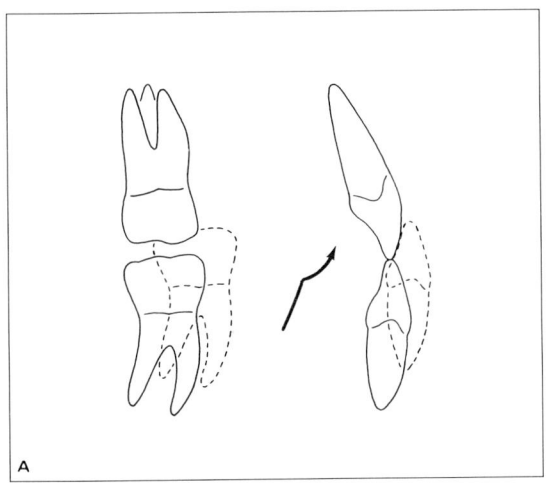 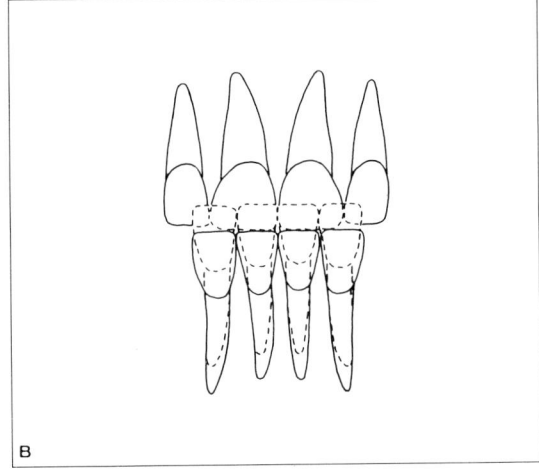

Fig. 14-4 Schematic presentation of an anterior forced bite, resulting in an anterior cross bite (progenic forced bite).

A   The initial contact is reached in the anterior region. After the ventral gliding movement, contact is attained in the posterior region.

B   Frontal view with initial contact and in maximal occlusion.

occlusion seems to exist. However, in a carefully directed closing movement in the most retruded mandibular position, initial contact is reached, for example, with the incisal edges of the maxillary lateral incisors followed by a gliding into anterior direction (Fig. 14-5). This type of anterior forced bite is easily overlooked. Anterior forced bites can also be based on unfavorable initial contacts of the posterior teeth.

Most forced bites are combinations of the anterior and lateral types. In forced bites, the position of the individual teeth adapts to the deviating maximal occlusion, with all variations that can occur in this respect.

Forced bites can be present in the deciduous dentition stage and in all later stages of the development of the dentition.

Occasionally, a situation is encountered in which a normal transverse relation exists on one side of the dental arch and a reversed one on the other. At a certain point on the dental arches, usually distally to the canines, the occlusal relation "crosses" (hence the name "cross bite") (Figs. 14-6 and 14-7). Cross bites may or may not be associated with lateral forced bites.

Total endo- or exo-occlusions of the posterior teeth with no contact at all between the occlusal surfaces are rare. A total exo-occlusion (Brodie syndrome[62]) is associated with a Class II/1 malocclusion (Fig. 14-8). Total endo-occlusions may occur in extreme Class III malocclusions (Fig. 14-9). The total endo- and exo-occlusions discussed here are sometimes called telescope bites.

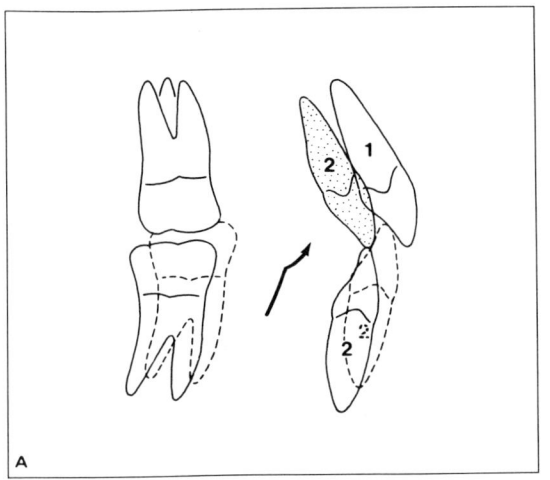 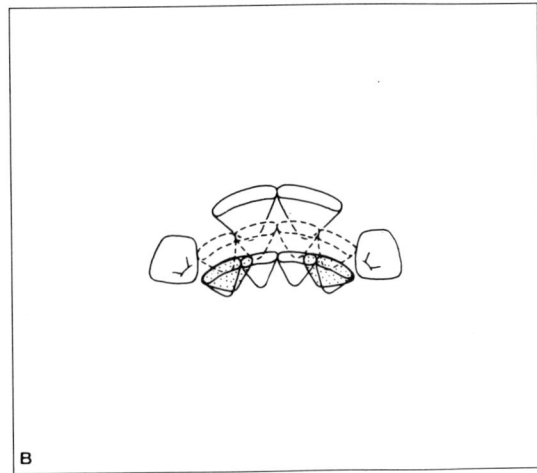

Fig. 14-5 Schematic presentation of an example of an anterior forced bite in a Class II/1 malocclusion, resulting in a situation that appears as a Class I in habitual occlusion.

A   In the normal closing movement of the mandible, initial contact is reached between the mandibular lateral permanent incisor and the maxillary one. From that position, the mandible glides ventrally and the mandibular lateral incisor becomes positioned between the lateral maxillary and central incisors. The molars attain a Class I occlusal relation.

B   Occlusal view of the maxillary four incisors and canines, drawn in combination with the mandibular four incisors in initial contact position (continuous lines) and after the ventral sliding movement (dotted lines). As in A, the maxillary lateral incisors have been meshed.

The situation illustrated here may occur in a Class II/1 malocclusion with considerable crowding in the maxillary dental arch. This is particularly true for cases in which the eruption and emergence of the maxillary central permanent incisors are associated with premature loss of the lateral deciduous incisors. Then, little or no increase of the intercanine distance is realized. The maxillary lateral permanent incisor will emerge palatally and, after attaining contact with the mandibular incisors, move further palatally. Subsequently, they may form the obstacle that leads to the protral gliding movement of the mandible.

Subdivisions, Forced Bites and Transverse Deviations

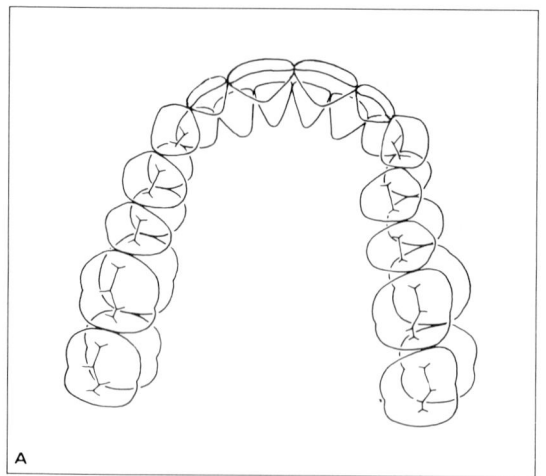 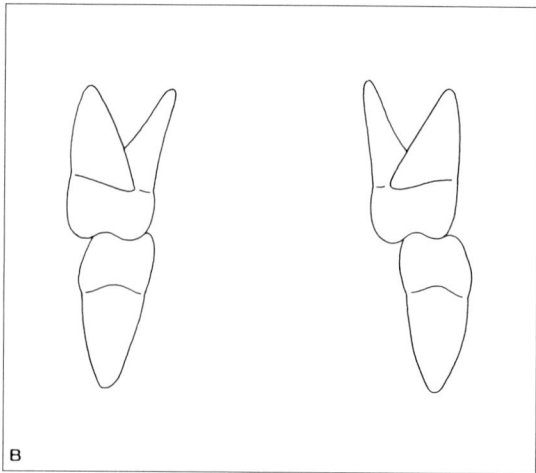

Fig. 14-6 Schematic presentation of a cross bite with a reversed transverse relation on one side.

A   The maxillary dental arch crosses the mandibular one distally to the maxillary left canine.
B   A normal transverse relation is present on the right side; an abnormal one on the left side.

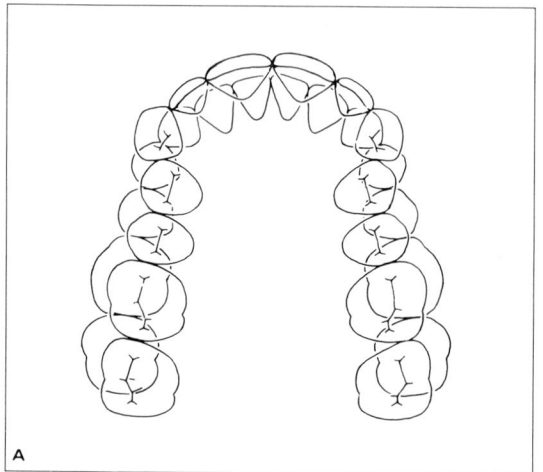 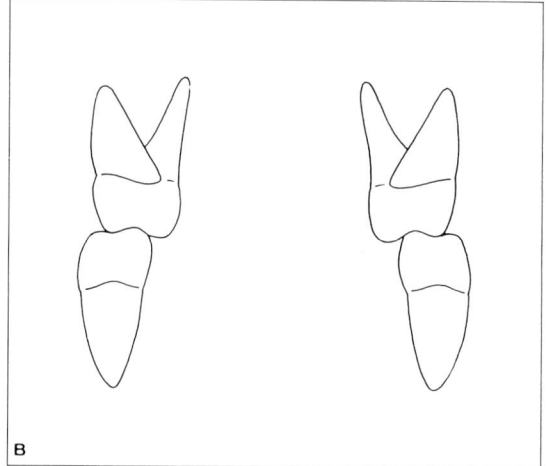

Fig. 14-7 Schematic presentation of a bilateral cross bite.

A   On both sides the maxillary posterior teeth occlude with their buccal cusps instead of their palatal ones.
B   Reversed transverse relation on both sides.

Subdivisions, Forced Bites and Transverse Deviations

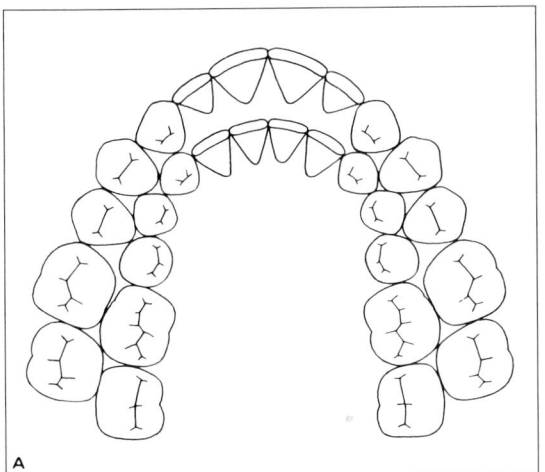 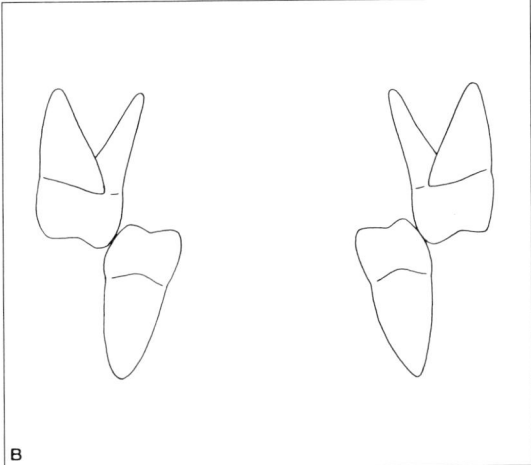

Fig. 14-8 Schematic presentation of an example of a total exo-occlusion in a Class II/1 malocclusion (Brodie syndrome).

A   The occlusal surfaces of the opposing posterior teeth do not make contact at all. All the maxillary teeth are positioned exteriorly to the mandibular ones (telescope bite).
B   As illustrated here for the first permanent molars, the maxillary posterior teeth are usually tipped buccally; the mandibular ones lingually.

Subdivisions, Forced Bites and Transverse Deviations

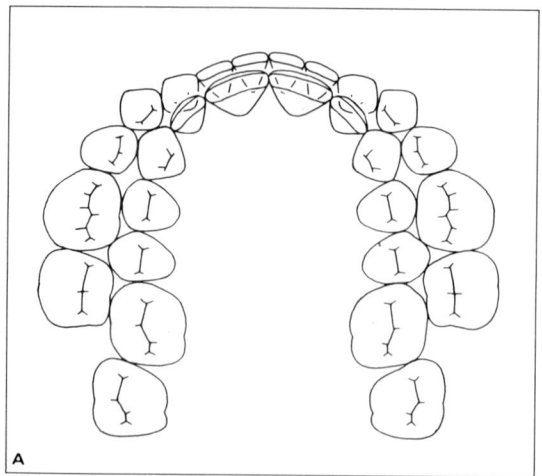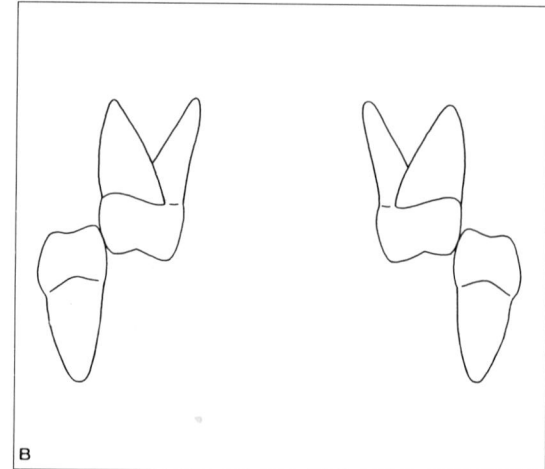

Fig. 14-9 Schematic presentation of an example of total endo-occlusion in a Class III malocclusion.

A   Nowhere does contact exist between the occlusal surfaces of the opposing posterior teeth. All the maxillary teeth are positioned interiorly to the mandibular ones.
B   The mandibular posterior teeth are usually buccally inclined; the maxillary ones lingually as illustrated here for the first permanent molars.

Endo-occlusion (as well as exo-occlusion) may occur partially. An anterior cross bite is an example of such a situation. An endo-occlusion may be limited to one side; it may also occur in the anterior region and only one posterior region.

Chapter 15

Results of Premature Loss of Deciduous Teeth

Deciduous teeth may be lost prematurely by trauma, premature resorption of their roots, decay, or by extraction. One of the most feared effects of premature loss is the migration of neighboring teeth into the space created. The successor of a prematurely lost tooth may find its space in the dental arch reduced or even fully lost. Although substantial loss of space in the dental arch will occur in many cases, it does not always happen by any means. The fear of the effects of premature loss of deciduous teeth is not always realistic. Loss from trauma is limited mainly to the maxillary incisors.

Resorption of roots of teeth, which normally should not yet be shed, may occur in crowded dental arches. Such resorption is mainly encountered in the mandibular and maxillary deciduous lateral incisors and canines. Once in a while it is seen in a maxillary second deciduous molar, when its distal root forms an obstacle to the eruption of the far mesially located adjacent first permanent molar.[10] Whether the deciduous molar will be shed prematurely depends, among other things, on the amount of root material that becomes resorbed.

Premature resorption of the root of a deciduous tooth usually occurs because the eruption of a permanent one is not only associated with the resorption of the root of its predecessor, but also with the one of an adjacent deciduous tooth. This is seen most frequently in the maxilla at the lateral deciduous incisor and in the mandible at the deciduous canine. A relatively large crown of an erupting maxillary central permanent incisor may lead not only to loss of the central deciduous incisor, but also of the lateral one. In the mandible, no median structure between the left and the right sides of the jaws is present after the first year of life. Crowding in the mandibular incisor region prior to emergence can result in an asymmetrical eruption pattern. Lack of space may be concentrated unilaterally and result in premature loss of one deciduous lateral incisor or one deciduous canine. The latter is the deciduous tooth that is most frequently lost as a result of premature root resorption in the mandible. In the maxilla, lack of space in the incisor region cannot be concentrated unilaterally in a corresponding manner, as the presence of the median intermaxillary suture acts as a barrier against a migration to the other side.

Further, deciduous canines are also the deciduous teeth most frequently lost due to premature extraction. Such extractions are intended to create space for a more favorable emergence of the lateral permanent incisors or to achieve a spontaneous improvement of the already emerged and malpositioned incisors. However, this procedure is indicated only under special conditions and should not be performed without careful consideration of the different aspects involved. Extraction of the deciduous canines may lead to situations that result in a less favorable subsequent development of the dentition than would otherwise have been the case.

Decay is the most common cause for premature loss of tooth material of deciduous molars. The mesiodistal crown dimension can become reduced and the available arch length may decrease.[27, 77] Decayed deciduous molars may loose their crowns partially or completely. Toothache or infections (alveolar fistulae) may lead to removal of roots and crown or of what has remained of them. Complete loss of deciduous molars due to decay, followed by extraction, occurs more than twice as often in the mandible as in the maxilla.[20, 42, 77, 99] Deciduous canines are more caries resistant than deciduous molars and rather seldom disappear for that reason. Deciduous incisors have only about half the infraoral lifetime as the other deciduous teeth and as such are less affected by decay.

The main results of premature loss of deciduous teeth are migrations of neighboring teeth toward the evoked diastema. These migrations depend on the tooth lost[19, 20, 40], the local conditions of occlusion,[20, 26, 56] and the sagittal relation between the two dental arches. The most important variable involved seems to be the spatial condition within the dental arch.[25, 26, 83] Also, the influence of the tongue and buccal musculature plays a role.[20, 42] Finally, the time of premature loss is essential.[25, 26] Premature loss long before the normal time of exfoliation seems to have a retarding effect on the eruption of the successor. Loss of a deciduous molar shortly prior to its normal time of exfoliation seems to have an accelerating effect on the eruption and emergence of its successor.[34]

In general, premature loss of deciduous teeth in subjects with an excess of dental arch space has a negligible effect or none at all on the subsequent development of the dentition and the ultimate location of the permanent teeth. In situations with no extra space available in the dental arches, premature loss of deciduous teeth may lead to several complications. Premature loss of deciduous teeth in crowded dental arches has almost always a distinctly unfavorable effect. As a rule, crowding will increase considerably.

Loss of deciduous molars prior to the emergence of first permanent molars as a rule has a larger negative effect than premature loss after the first permanent molars have attained occlusion. In the former case, the crowns of the second premolars are relatively far away from the occlusal plane and as such play a lesser role in the prevention of mesial drift of the first permanent molars than when they are situated more occlusally. Further, a first permanent molar tends to emerge earlier and more mesially when the adjacent deciduous molar is no longer present.[26, 86] Premature loss of deciduous molars prior to the emergence of the second permanent molars will result in a more mesial migration of the first permanent molars than in the reversed situation.[53, 103] Further, in cases with premature loss of deciduous molars, the emergence of the second permanent molars in those quadrants is advanced.[86]

In general, early premature loss of deciduous teeth has a larger negative impact on the subsequent development of the dentition than late premature loss. Migrations that occur as a result of premature loss mainly take place within the first 6 months following the loss.[83] In the maxilla, the migrations are more extensive and occur more rapidly than in the mandible.[20, 78, 85] Furthermore, in the maxilla, the migrations are mainly limited to mesial displacements of the permanent first molars, while in the mandible, the teeth mesial to the diastema tend to move distally in addition.[78] However, frequently the loss of space is limited and often negligible.[19, 26, 40, 53, 56, 80, 90] In many cases, the initial reduction of space is substantially regained during the later part of the mixed dentition period.[58]

The results of premature loss of deciduous teeth are predictable; however, this is not always a simple task. Many variables have to be taken into account in such a prediction procedure. The variables involved and the reasoning behind them will be treated mainly on the basis of schematic drawings. Most attention in this respect will be paid to the loss of the second deciduous molars, as these are the key teeth in premature loss. The effects of premature loss of the first deciduous molars is comparable to those of the second ones however, they are less severe.[20, 40] On the basis of the information supplied about premature loss of the second deciduous molars, the effect of the premature loss of the first molars can be estimated.

In the maxillary anterior region, premature loss is usually caused by trauma. In the deciduous dentition, one or two maxillary central incisors are most frequently involved. An intruding movement of a maxillary central deciduous incisor may result in a displacement of the superiorly located crown of the corresponding central permanent incisor. Delayed emergence or no spontaneous emergence at all of the latter may be the result. The situation is even worse when the inclination of the permanent tooth germ becomes changed. As a result, the crown may attain an abnormal position, usually a more or less horizontal one with its incisal edge directed ventrally. The formation of the tooth is completed in the original setting. The crown may become misshapen. However, in most instances, trauma takes place after root formation of the permanent central incisor has already commenced. The deviation in the tooth will then be located at the root.

No—or only slight—displacement of the central permanent incisor occurs when the trauma does not involve an intruding movement of its predecessor. This is frequently the case when the deciduous central incisor is lost in an accident, as often happens in the last phase of the complete deciduous dentition stage. Then the consequences of the trauma are generally limited to a more labial eruption and emergence of the central permanent incisor involved and a considerable delay in its piercing of the gingival tissue—often more than one year.[48] The presence of the maxillary central deciduous incisors is not essential in the maintenance of space for their successors in the dental arch. Further, maxillary central deciduous incisors do not play a role, like the lateral ones, in the increase of the transverse intercanine distance (Fig. 15-1A). A maxillary lateral deciduous incisor is most frequently lost prematurely by too early resorption of its root in association with the eruption of the adjacent central permanent incisor. As has been explained, this type of premature loss usually takes place only in cases of crowding. It often occurs bilaterally (Fig. 15-1B). After premature loss

Results of Premature Loss of Deciduous Teeth

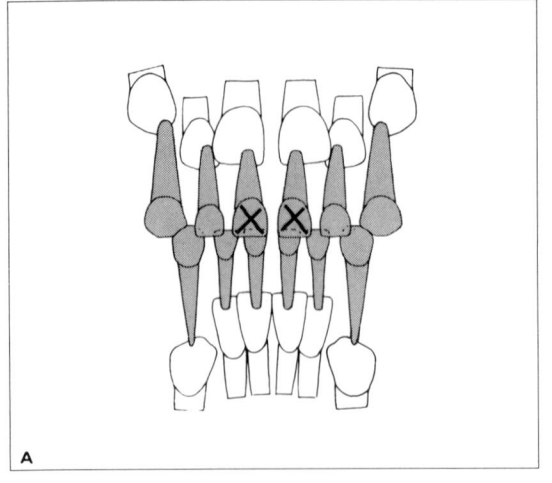
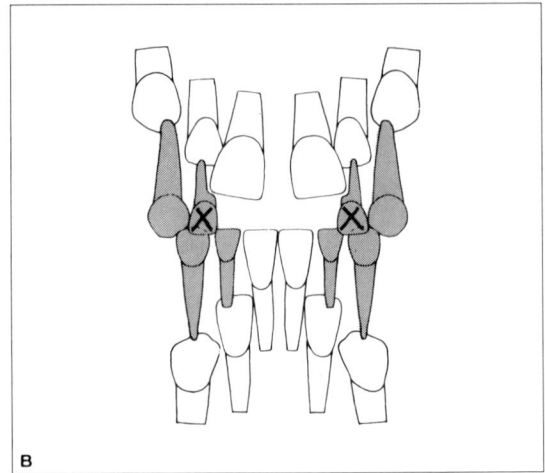
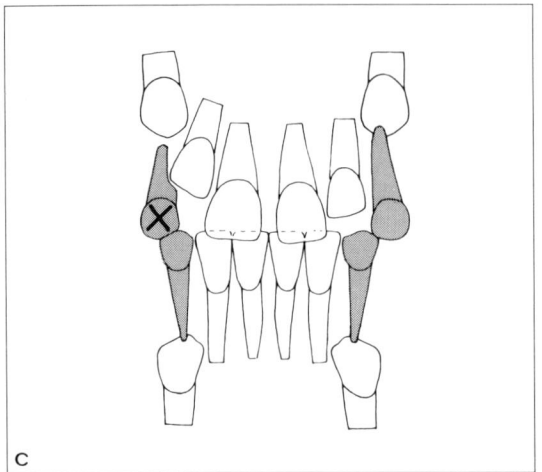
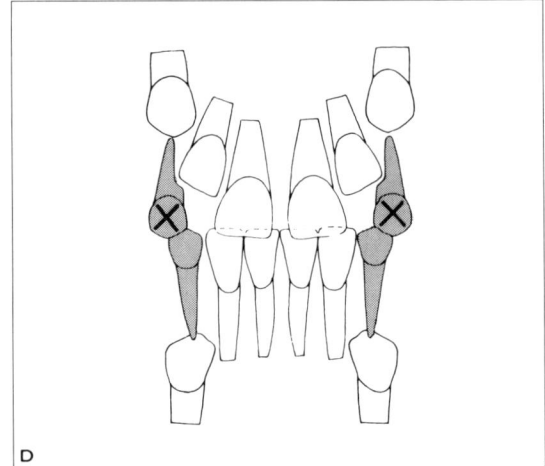

Fig. 15-1 Schematic illustrations to clarify the effect of premature loss of maxillary deciduous incisors and canines.

A Trauma to the maxillary deciduous incisors can lead to loss of the central ones and to disturbances in the formation, position, eruption, and emergence of their successors, particularly of maxillary central permanent incisors. Otherwise, the development of the dentition is not affected when only maxillary central deciduous incisors are lost.

B Premature loss of both maxillary lateral deciduous incisors due to early resorption in a case of crowding. The maxillary deciduous intercanine distance increase associated with the eruption of the central permanent incisors can be no longer attained.

C Premature loss of the maxillary right deciduous canine during eruption of the maxillary right lateral permanent incisor. Subsequently, the four maxillary permanent incisors will migrate into the direction of the premature loss. Accordingly, the midpoints of the mandibular and maxillary dental arch will change in relation. A midline deviation will develop.

D Premature loss of both maxillary deciduous canines.

of a maxillary lateral deciduous incisor, the deciduous canine on that side will not become displaced laterally during the eruption of the maxillary central permanent incisor in the way explained in Chapter 4. In cases of bilateral premature loss of maxillary lateral deciduous incisors, the intercanine distance does not increase. After unilateral premature loss, both maxillary central permanent incisor crowns will migrate in the direction where the extra space in the dental arch has become available. This movement will result in a discordance of the medians of the two dental arches. The maxillary and mandibular contact points between the central incisors or the midpoints of the central diastema will no longer match. The dentition shows midline deviation. The eruption of a maxillary lateral permanent incisor may be associated with premature loss of the adjacent deciduous canine in a similar way as indicated above (Figs. 15-1C and D). Unilateral premature loss will be followed by migration of the four maxillary permanent incisors toward the site of the loss. A midline deviation will result. Later, insufficient space will be available for the permanent canine in the dental arch, which will emerge in a buccal position and become located outside the dental arch. Bilateral premature loss of deciduous canines in crowding usually will lead to buccal position of both maxillary permanent canines.

Premature loss of mandibular deciduous incisors may occur under comparable circumstances. However, traumata seldom involve mandibular deciduous incisors. Premature loss of a mandibular lateral deciduous incisor usually takes place unilaterally (Fig.15-2A) and often is associated with an asymmetrical position and emergence of the four mandibular permanent incisors. The same holds true for unilateral loss of a mandibular deciduous canine (Fig. 15-2C). Bilateral loss of mandibular lateral deciduous incisors (Fig. 15-2B) or canines (Fig. 15-2D) occurs less frequently than unilateral loss. The lateral displacement of the mandibular deciduous canine, which may take place during the eruption of the mandibular central permanent incisor in cases with crowding, cannot occur if the lateral deciduous incisor is lost prematurely.

Premature loss of maxillary and mandibular deciduous incisors and canines may be followed by changes in the size of the overjet and overbite. These changes will be treated at the end of this chapter.

In the discussion of premature loss of deciduous molars, a differentiation is made between normal anteroposterior dental arch relations, Class II, and Class III malocclusions. As indicated above, sagittal occlusal relations between individual teeth play an essential role in the effect that may result from premature loss.

As already noted, premature loss of second deciduous molars will be treated extensively. Relatively little attention will be paid to premature loss of first deciduous molars. The principles involved in the prediction of the results of premature loss of deciduous molars are more or less the same for the first and the second ones. However, a distinct difference in the effects of the premature loss of first and second deciduous molars regards the migration of adjacent teeth. The eventual migration after premature loss of a second deciduous molar will mainly be restricted to mesial migration of the first permanent molar, particularly in the maxilla. After premature loss of the first deciduous molar, an eventual reduction of space is likely to occur as well

Results of Premature Loss of Deciduous Teeth

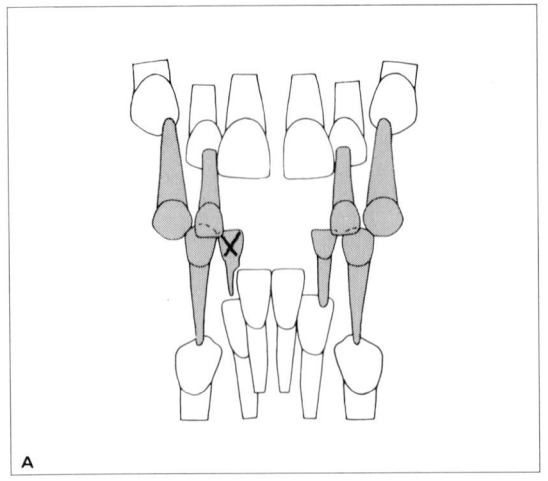
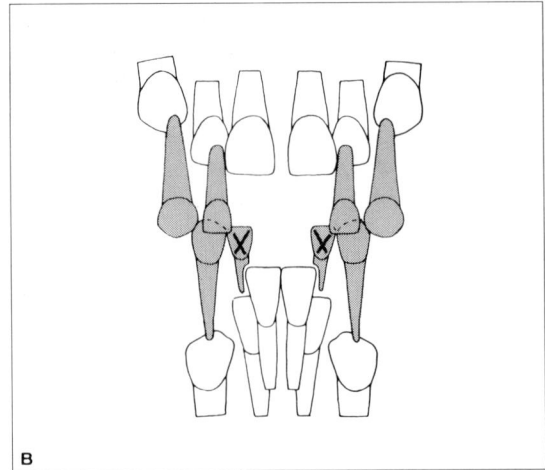
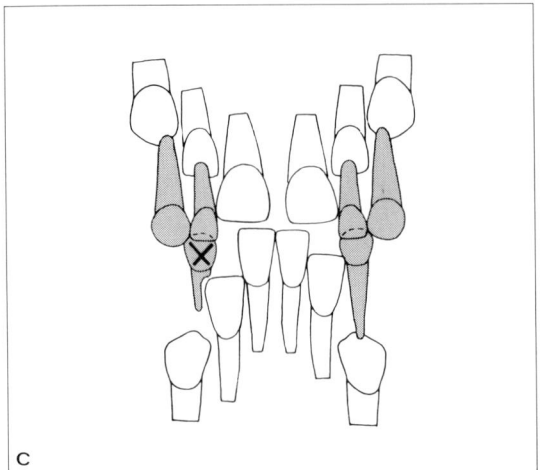
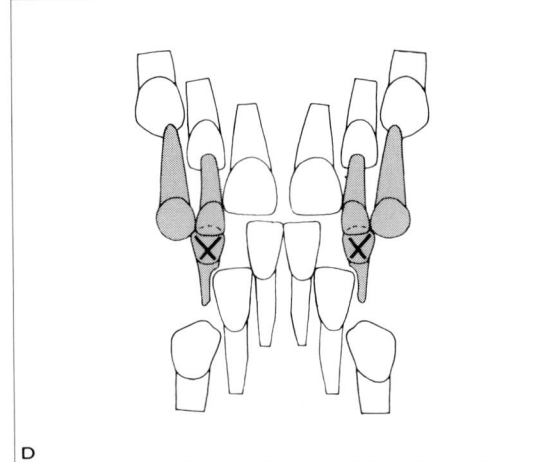

Fig. 15-2 Premature loss of mandibular lateral deciduous incisors and canines.

A   Unilateral loss of one mandibular lateral deciduous incisor, as may happen in cases with an asymmetrical orientation and eruption of the mandibular permanent incisors.
B   The same bilaterally. The distance between the two mandibular deciduous canines will not increase in association with the eruption of the mandibular central permanent incisors.
C   Unilateral loss of a mandibular deciduous canine, which will be followed by migration of the mandibular permanent incisors and midline deviation.
D   The same bilaterally; as a rule, with no midline deviation.

by distal migration of mesially located teeth, particularly in the mandible. As previously indicated, the second deciduous molar is a key tooth regarding premature loss and its loss has greater impact on the subsequent development of the dentition than that of the first deciduous molar.[20,40]

It is repeated here that mesial migration of the first permanent molar generally involves an acceleration of the eruption of the adjacent second permanent molar and an advancement of its time of emergence.

Again, it is stated explicitly that premature loss of deciduous teeth by no means always results in permanent adverse effects. The space available later in the dental arch for the permanent teeth may still be adequate. Not only may the migration that occurs subsequent to the premature loss be minimal and negligible, but also space reduced due to migration following premature loss can eventually be regained.[58]

In patients with sufficient dental arch space and normal occlusal relations, premature loss of mandibular second deciduous molars seldom will lead to problems. This is contrary to the situation in the maxilla, as premature loss of maxillary second deciduous molars usually results in adverse effects. The difference in this respect between the two jaws is based on three phenomena. First, the mandibular deciduous molar generally has a larger mesiodistal crown width than the maxillary one. In normal anteroposterior dental arch relations (Class I), a flush terminal plane exists. On premature loss of the mandibular second deciduous molar, the maxillary one will overerupt and in its supraposition act as a barrier against mesial migration of the mandibular first permanent molar beyond its cuspal interference (Fig. 15-3). The occlusal relations determine if and when this barrier phenomenon will take place. The course of the terminal plane is essential in this respect.

In cases of premature loss of a maxillary second deciduous molar, a comparable situation cannot develop, as the mandibular second deciduous molar with its larger mesiodistal crown dimension cannot overerupt. The mandibular second deciduous molar has not only one, but two antagonists: the maxillary first deciduous molar also occludes with it (Fig. 15-4). Subsequent to the premature loss of the maxillary second deciduous molar, the maxillary first permanent molar can migrate mesially. This migration is not a parallel one, but involves a rotation around the axis through the mesiopalatal cusp and the palatal root. This cusp happens to occlude in the central fossa of the mandibular first permanent molar. The palatal root is the largest and longest root of the maxillary first permanent molar.

Premature loss of the second deciduous molars in both jaws at the same time almost always has an adverse effect on the subsequent development of the dentition (Fig. 15-5). Mesial migration of the mandibular first permanent molar can no longer be blocked by an overerupted maxillary second deciduous molar. Both the mandibular and maxillary first permanent molars migrate mesially. The maxillary one migrates more than it would have done if the premature loss had taken place only in the maxilla. With the mesial migration of the mandibular first permanent molar, its central fossa drifts anteriorly and no longer serves as a point of resistance against the mesial migration of the maxillary first permanent molar.

The second phenomenon in which the two jaws differ regarding the permanent effect of premature loss of deciduous teeth is in the potential of remigration of mesially displaced first permanent molars. Mandibular first permanent molars have a large

Results of Premature Loss of Deciduous Teeth

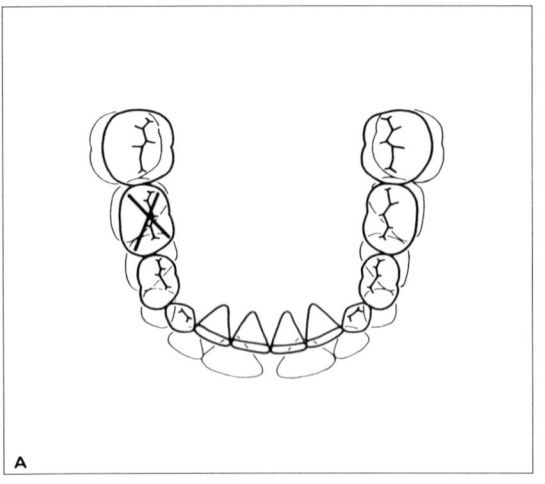
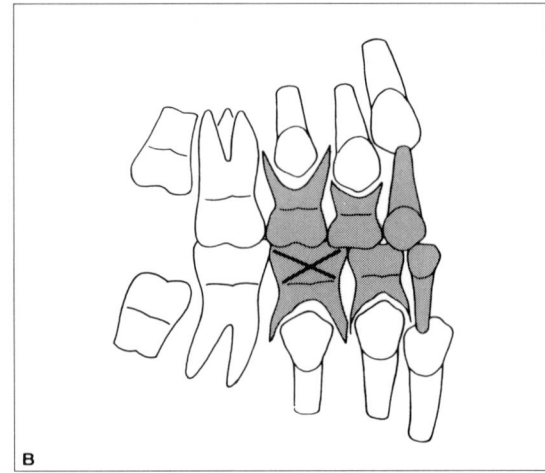
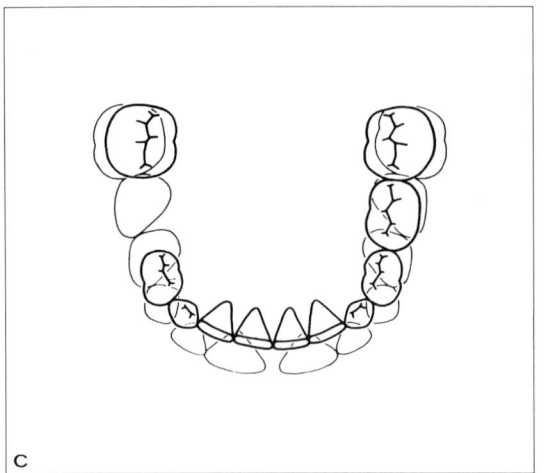
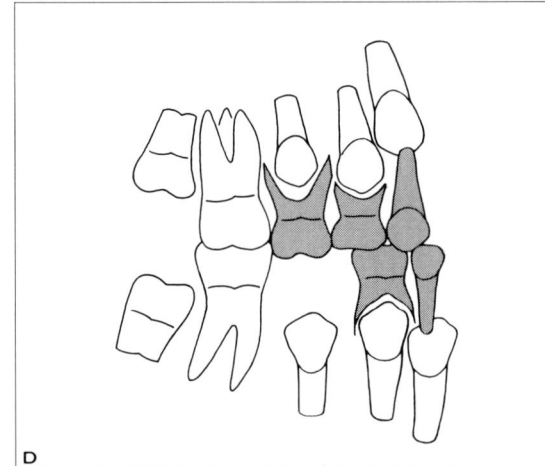

Fig. 15-3   Premature loss of the mandibular right second deciduous molar in a Class I situation.

A,B   The mandibular second deciduous molar has a larger mesiodistal crown dimension than the maxillary one. Accordingly, the terminal plane of the deciduous dentition has only a small mesial step.

C,D   The maxillary second deciduous molar can overerupt and in supraposition act as a barrier against mesial migration of the mandibular right first permanent molar. The subsequent development of the dentition will not experience adverse results from the premature loss.

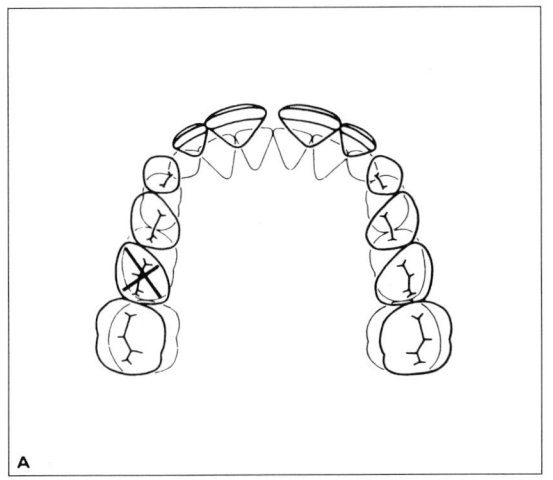 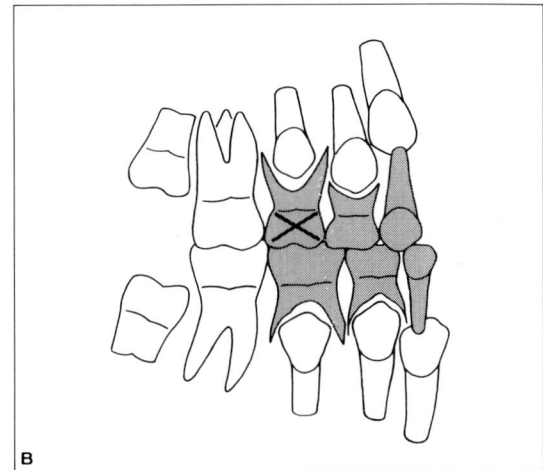
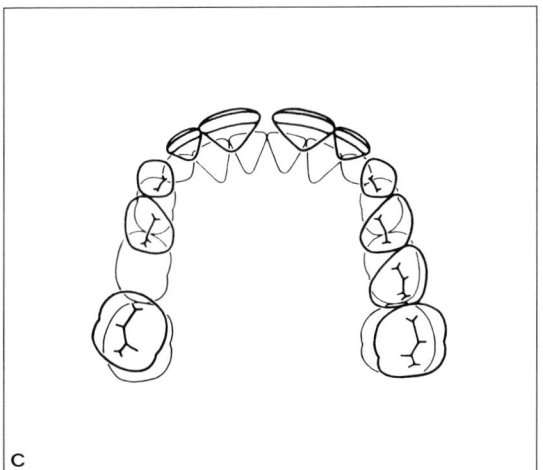 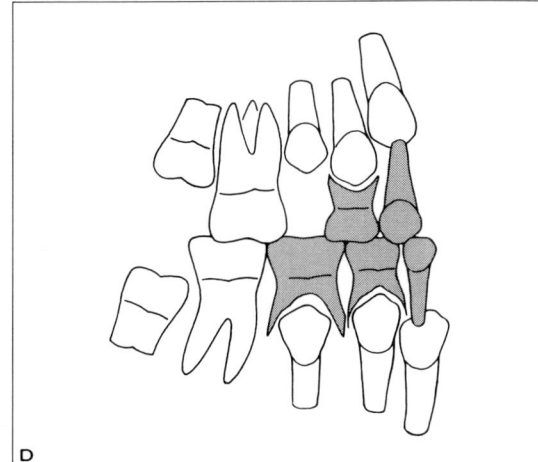

Fig. 15-4 Premature loss of the maxillary right second deciduous molar in a Class I situation.

A,B The mandibular second deciduous molar has a larger mesiodistal crown dimension than the maxillary one. Consequently, it occludes with two maxillary teeth. After premature loss of the maxillary second deciduous molar, the first one still will prevent an overeruption of the mandibular second deciduous molar.

C,D The maxillary right first permanent molar migrates mesially and rotates around an axis through the mesiopalatal cusp and the palatal root. The rotational movement results in a considerable loss of space as the maxillary first permanent molar has a rhomboid-shaped crown.

Results of Premature Loss of Deciduous Teeth

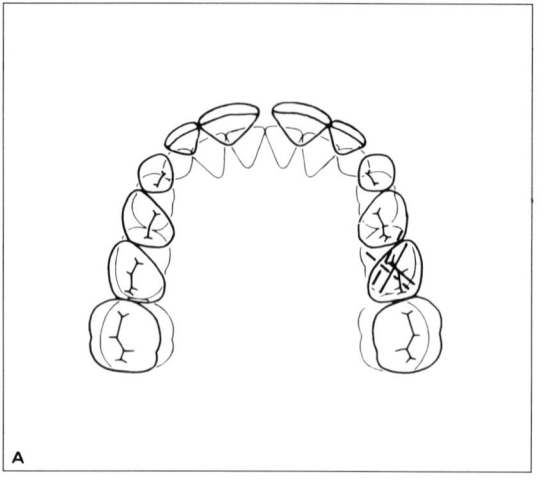
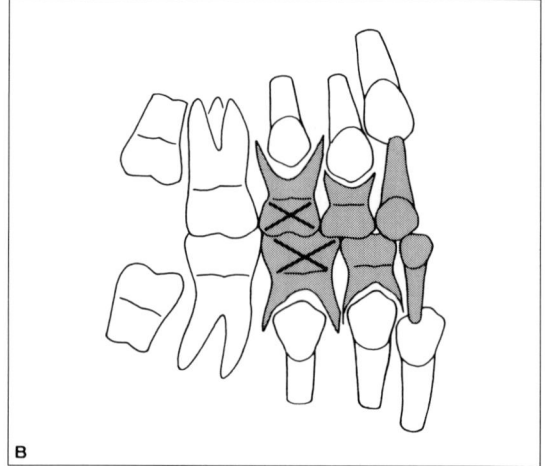
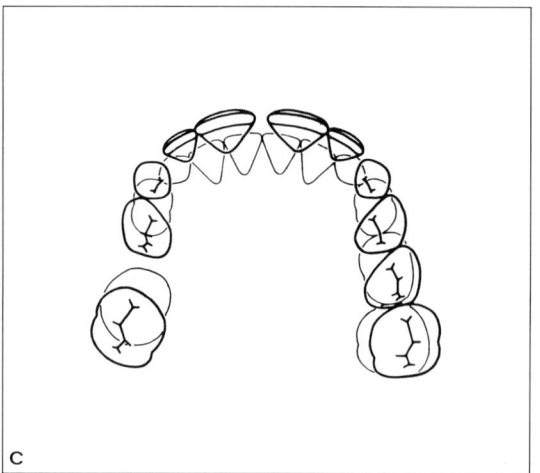
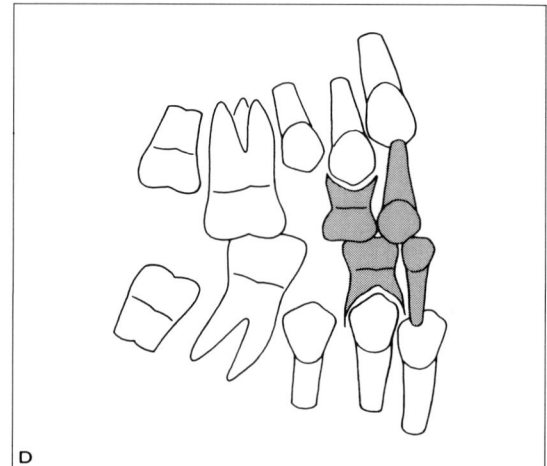

Fig. 15-5 Unilateral premature loss of mandibular and maxillary second deciduous molars in a Class I situation.

A,B After premature loss of both second deciduous molars on one side, the mesial migration of the mandibular first permanent molar will not be blocked by the overerupted second deciduous molar.

C,D The mandibular and maxillary first permanent molars migrate mesially. The maxillary one migrates more than it would have if only the maxillary second deciduous molar were lost. The mesial displacement of the mandibular first permanent molar is also often accompanied by a slight mesiolingual rotation.

Mesial migration of first permanent molars after premature loss of deciduous molars may result in an accelerated eruption and advanced emergence of the second permanent molars.

potential in this respect; maxillary ones have a limited potential. During the eruption and emergence of the mandibular second premolars, the first permanent molars which previously had migrated mesially may become displaced distally. Reduced available space caused by distal migration of mesially located teeth may be regained. The limited potential in regaining lost space in the maxilla is related to the rhomboid-shaped morphology of the maxillary first permanent molar crown. Consequently, the space between the now emerged first premolar and the rotated maxillary first permanent molar becomes trapezoid in configuration. The erupting maxillary second premolar finds its space for emergence reduced and will go for the way of least resistance and deviate palatally. The force exerted by the erupting maxillary second premolar in distal direction on the adjacent first permanent molar will have little or no effect on the location of the latter. The situation in the mandible is different, as the first permanent molar migrates mesially in a more or less parallel movement. In addition, its mesial surface is almost flat and oriented nearly perpendicularly to the direction of the dental arch. It is not only on the basis of mechanical grounds that the mandibular second premolar can regain the lost space that was originally intended for this tooth in the dental arch. With regard to jaw shape and bone structure, more favorable conditions for regaining space exist in the mandible than in the maxilla. The trapezoid configuration in the maxilla (indicated above) consists not so much of compact as of spongy bone.

The third phenomenon that leads to a more favorable result in the mandible than in the maxilla after premature loss of deciduous molars lies in the difference in the sum of the mesiodistal crown dimensions of the first and second deciduous molars compared to those of their predecessors. This difference is larger for the mandibular than for the maxillary teeth. More space can be lost in the mandible than in the maxilla before a problem arises. This particularly holds true in conditions in which much space is available for the teeth in the mandibular dental arch.

The effects of premature loss of deciduous molars in Class II/1 malocclusions are different from those in normal situations because the occlusion differs. In addition, other factors play a role. Of special importance are the typical relations between lips and teeth that accompany Class II/1 malocclusions. The lower lip usually exerts a more lingually directed pressure on the mandibular incisors than in normal situations. The maxillary incisors may undergo labially directed force, particularly when the lower lip is positioned in rest and during functional activity palatally to the maxillary incisors.

Premature loss of a mandibular second deciduous molar in a Class II/1 malocclusion is not followed by overeruption of the maxillary one as the latter also occludes with the mandibular first deciduous molar. The mesial migration of the mandibular first permanent molar is not confined by an extruded maxillary second deciduous molar (Fig. 15-6). Further, the extraction space can become reduced even more by additional distal migration of the mesially located teeth.

In a Class II/1 malocclusion, the maxillary first permanent molar also migrates and rotates mesially after premature loss of the maxillary second deciduous molar (Fig. 15-7).

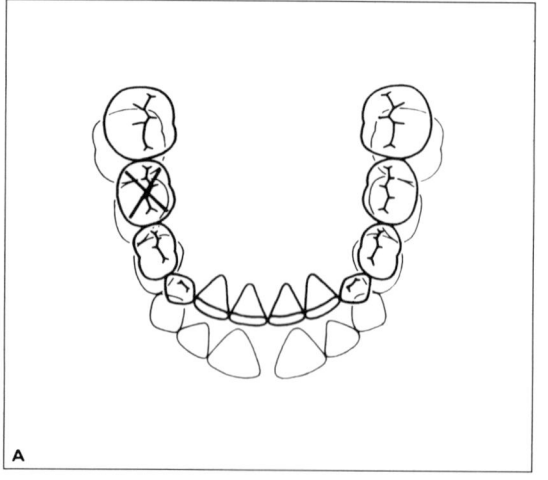 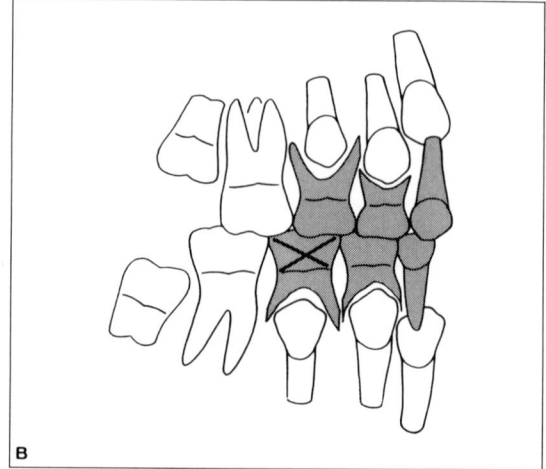
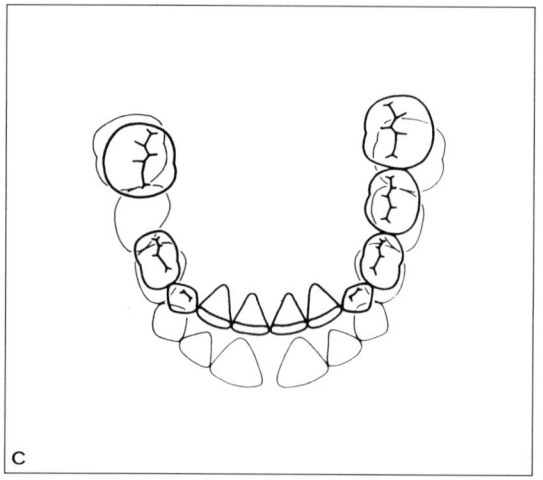 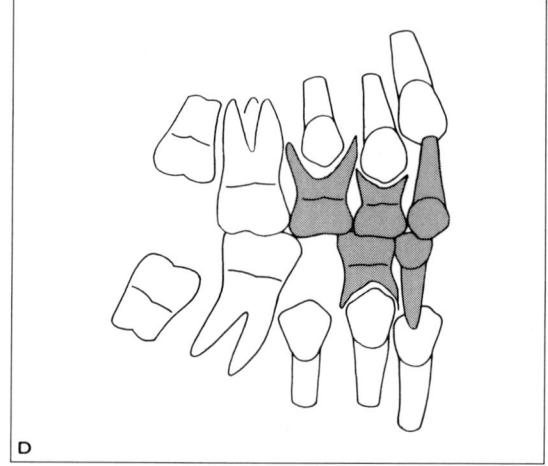

Fig. 15-6 Premature loss of the mandibular right deciduous molar in a Class II/1 malocclusion.

A,B The maxillary second deciduous molar does not occlude only with the mandibular second one, but with the mandibular first one as well.

C,D As the maxillary second deciduous molar cannot overerupt, no blocking of the mesial migration of the mandibular first permanent molar can take place. If the lower lip is positioned between the mandibular and maxillary incisors, the space created in the dental arch will become reduced more by distal migration of the mesially positioned teeth than otherwise would have been the case.

Results of Premature Loss of Deciduous Teeth

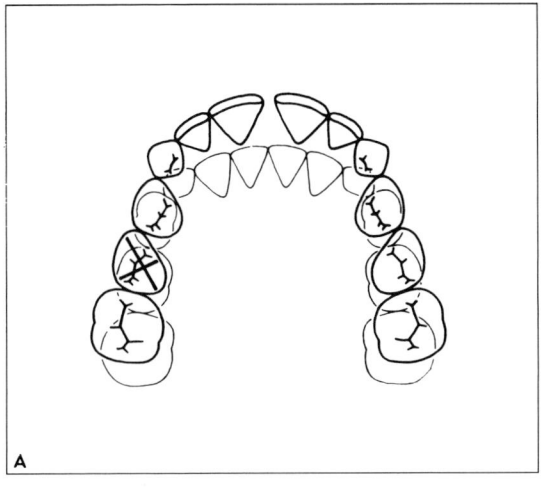
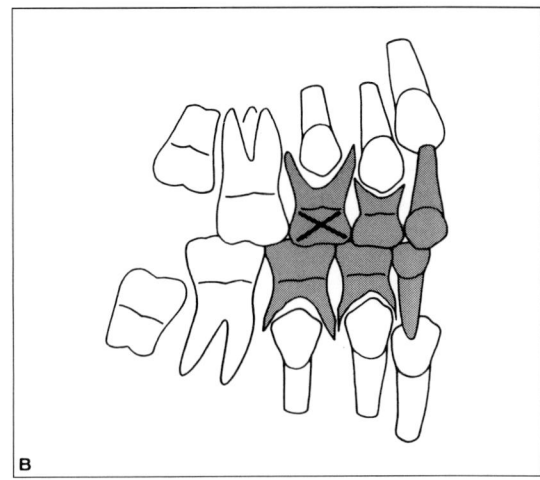
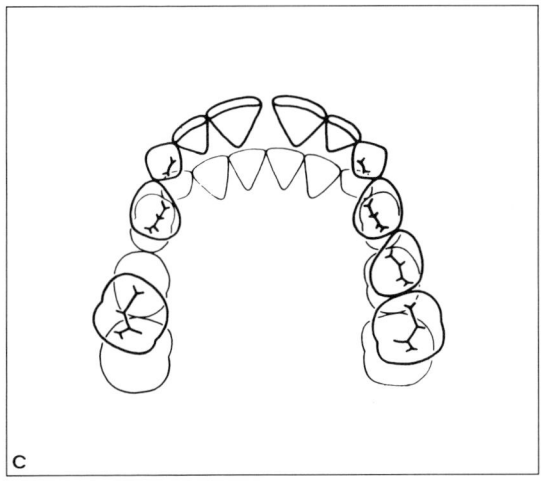
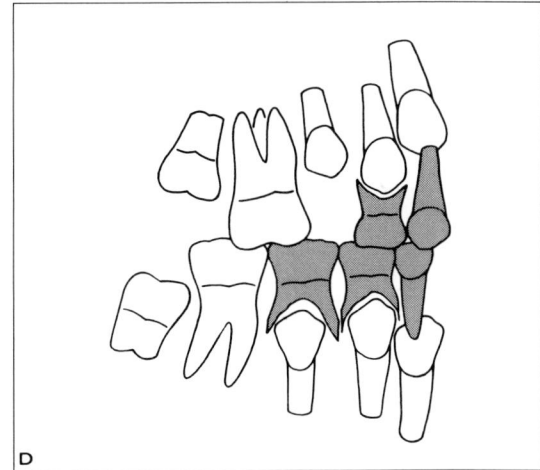

Fig. 15-7 Premature loss of the maxillary right second deciduous molar in a Class II/1 malocclusion.

A,B Also under these conditions, the mesiodistally large mandibular second deciduous molar cannot overerupt.
C,D The maxillary first permanent molar migrates and rotates mesially. Its mesiopalatal cusp does not occlude in the central fossa of the mandibular first permanent molar and as such there is less restriction in mesial migration by occlusion.

Results of Premature Loss of Deciduous Teeth

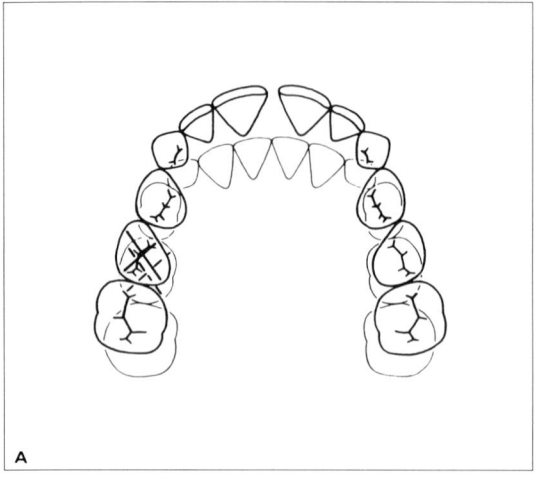
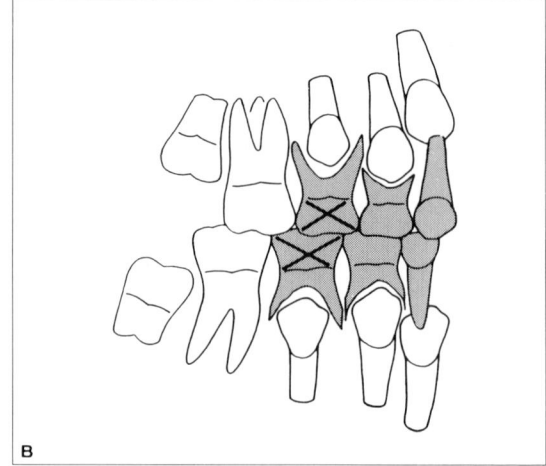
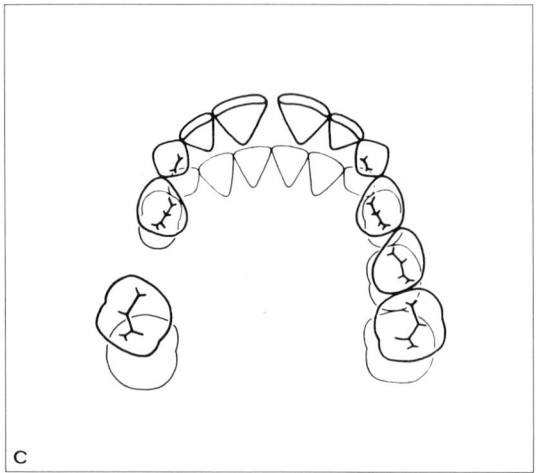
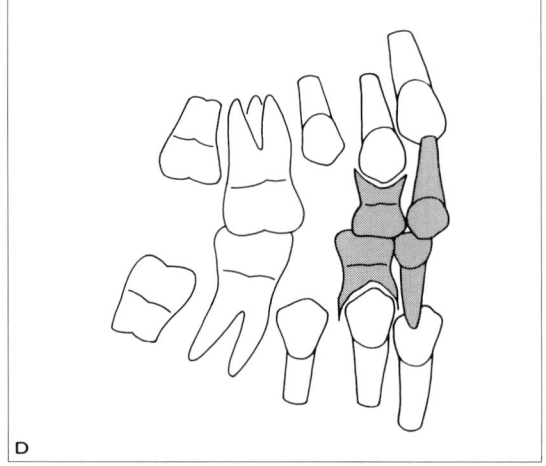

Fig. 15-8   Unilateral premature loss of the mandibular and maxillary second deciduous molars in a Class II/1 malocclusion.

A,B *After premature loss of both second deciduous molars on one side, no overeruption takes place.*

C,D *The mandibular and maxillary first permanent molars migrate mesially. Often the mesial migration is larger in the mandibular than in the maxillary arch, in accordance with the larger mesiodistal crown dimension of the lost mandibular second deciduous molar than that of the maxillary.*

If the mandibular and the maxillary second deciduous molars are lost prematurely unilaterally, the adjacent first permanent molars in both jaws will migrate mesially (Fig. 15-8). The loss of space is usually larger in the mandible than in the maxilla because, among other things, the difference in mesiodistal crown dimensions between the deciduous and permanent teeth is larger in the mandible than in the maxilla. More important, however, is the distal migration of the mesially located teeth, which may easily occur in Class II/1 malocclusions. Detrimental is premature loss of all four mandibular deciduous molars in a Class II/1 malocclusion with the lower lip positioned between the maxillary and mandibular incisors as the latter may easily move lingually when the first deciduous molars are missing. Consequently, the space for the premolars may become reduced (Fig. 15-9), as may happen particularly with crowding in the mandibular dental arch.

In Class II/2 malocclusions, the tendency for distal migration of the teeth positioned mesially to the premature extraction site will be extra large. Premature loss of mandibular deciduous molars may result in an increase of the lingual tipping of the mandibular and maxillary incisors. Premature loss of deciduous molars and canines in both jaws is especially unfavorable. Regarding the other aspects related to premature loss of deciduous teeth, the conditions are more or less comparable to those described above for Class II/1 malocclusions.

In a Class III malocclusion with an anterior cross bite, not the mandibular incisors but the maxillary ones will tend to tip lingually after premature loss of deciduous molars. The effects of premature loss of deciduous molars in Class III malocclusions are elaborated on in Figures 15-10 through 15-13.

The results of premature loss of deciduous molars have been discussed and illustrated for the normal sagittal dental arch relation and for Class II/1 and Class III malocclusions of one full premolar crown width. However, many cases with premature loss have occlusal relations that do not conform exactly to one of these three conditions, but are somewhere in between. Every individual instance has to be judged by its own merits. The prediction of a specific premature loss has to be performed on the basis of quite a few variables, among which are the occlusal relations. This discussion is intended to explain the principles involved and focus on those variables most essential in arriving at an adequate evaluation of the situation and a dependable prediction. By presenting the fundamentals regarding the factors of importance in premature loss, the changes that subsequently may take place, and above all whether these changes will or will not effect the ultimate situation of the permanent dentition in an adverse way, it is hoped that readers will be able to arrive at a valid judgment in the situations they will encounter.

Finally, some remarks may be made regarding the effect of premature loss of deciduous teeth on the transverse relation between the midpoints of the mandibular and maxillary dental arches and on the overjet and overbite.
Unilateral loss of a maxillary deciduous canine leads to a tipping of the four maxillary incisors in the direction where the loss took place. This change in angulation is

Results of Premature Loss of Deciduous Teeth

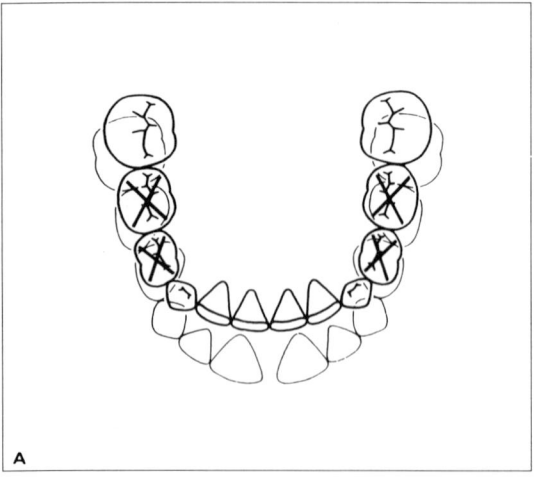
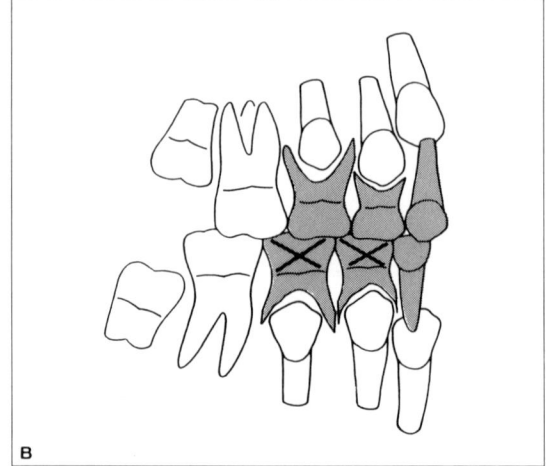
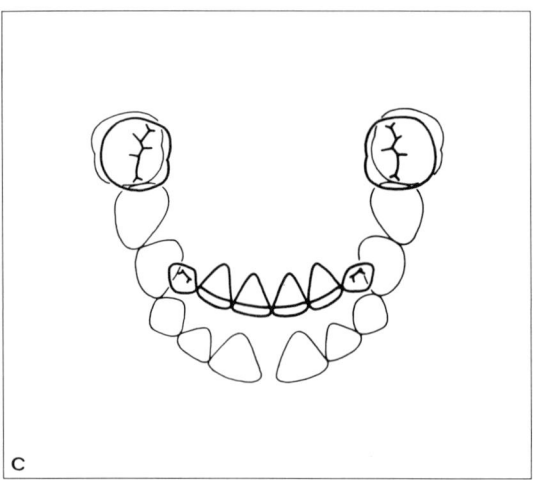
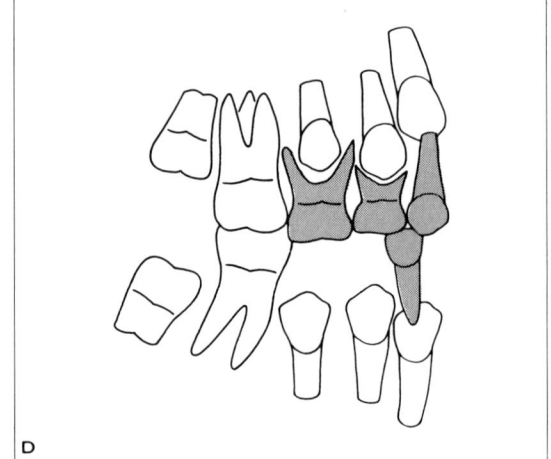

Fig. 15-9 Bilateral premature loss of the mandibular first and second deciduous molars in a Class II/1 malocclusion.

A,B The maxillary second deciduous molars can overerupt because not only the mandibular second but also the mandibular first deciduous molars are lost.

C,D The mandibular first permanent molars migrate mesially until they are blocked by the overerupted second deciduous molars. The space in the mandible is further substantially reduced by lingual tipping of the mandibular incisors under the influence of forces exerted by the lower lip.

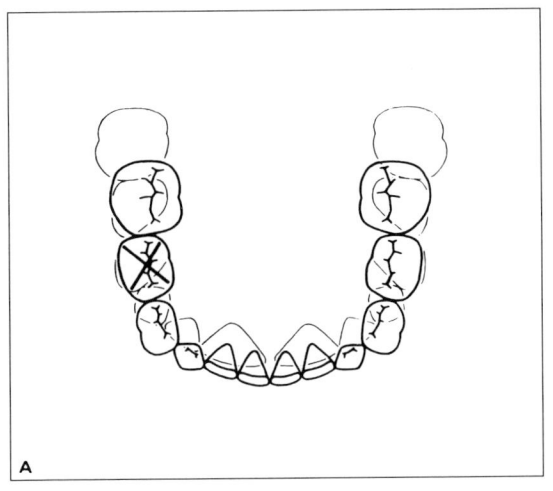 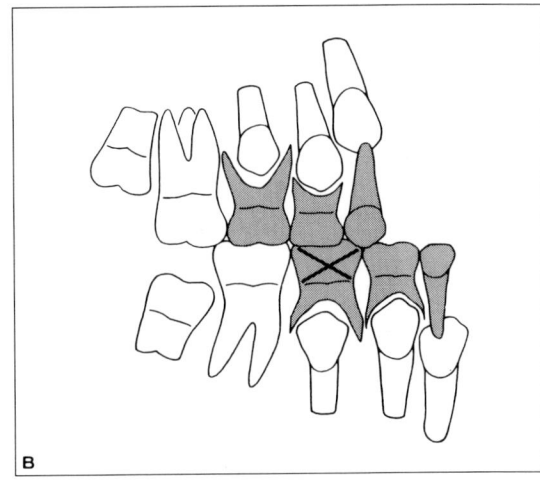

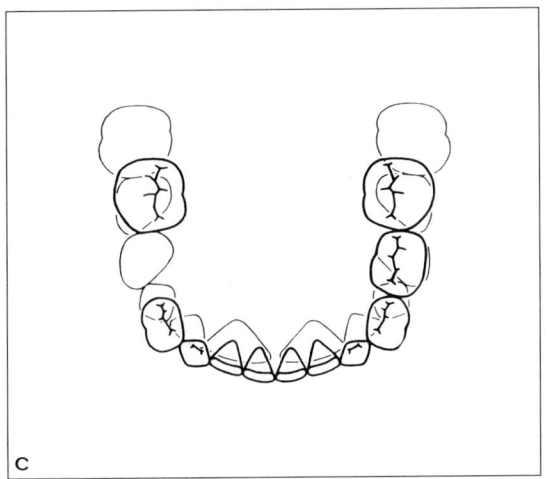 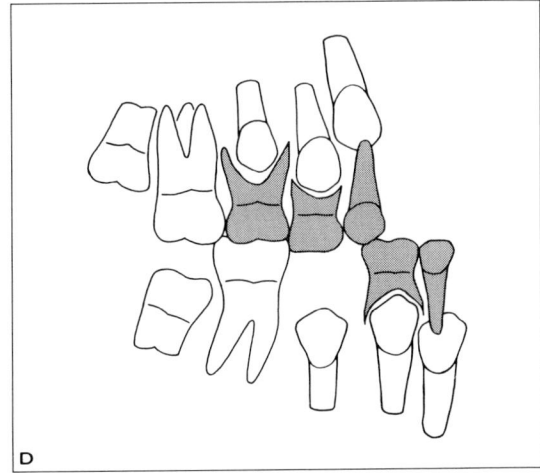

Fig. 15-10 Premature loss of the mandibular right second deciduous molar in a Class III malocclusion.

A,B The maxillary first deciduous molar can overerupt in the space provided after premature loss of the mandibular second deciduous molar.
C,D The mandibular first permanent molar migrates only slightly; the overerupted maxillary first deciduous molar acts as a barrier against further mesial migration.

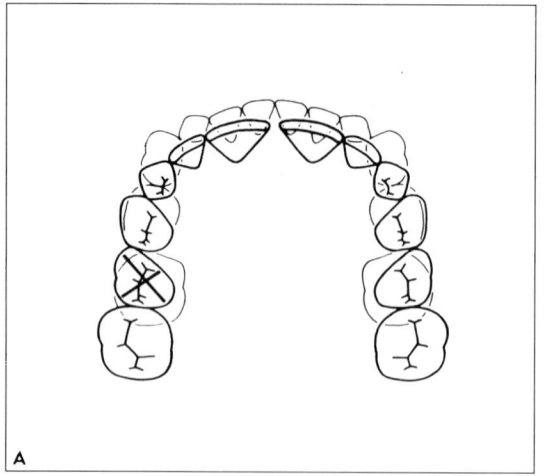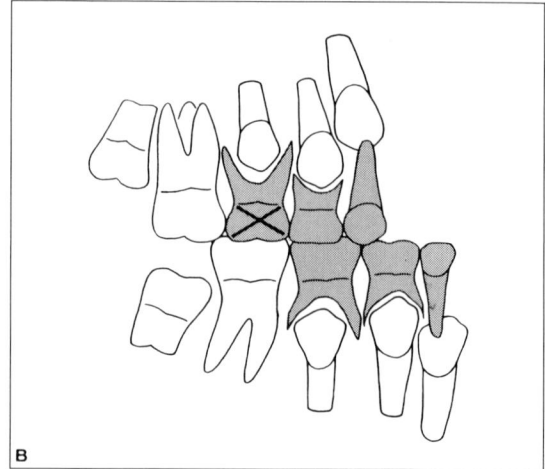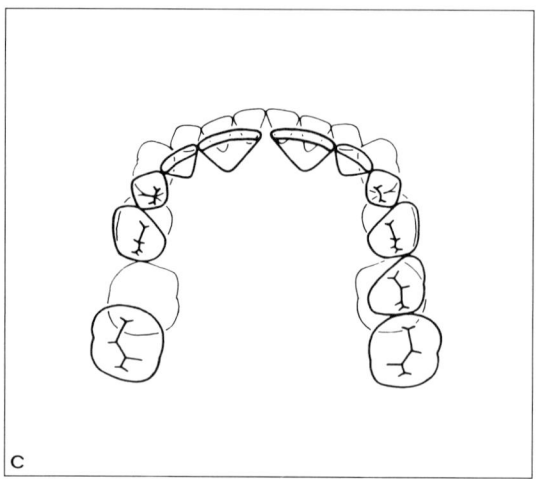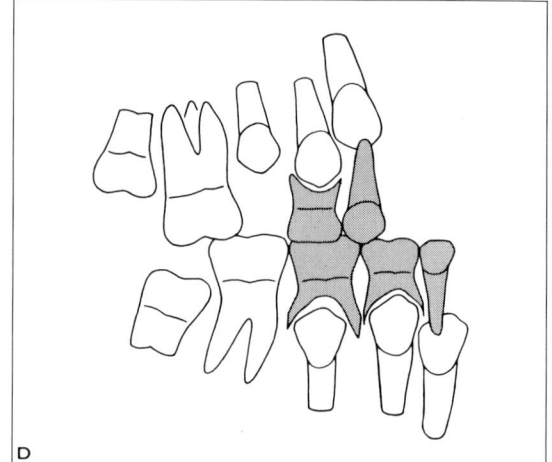

Fig. 15-11 Premature loss of a maxillary right second deciduous molar in a Class III malocclusion.

A,B No possibility for overeruption of a mandibular deciduous molar after the premature loss in the maxilla.

C,D The maxillary first permanent molar migrates and rotates mesially.

Results of Premature Loss of Deciduous Teeth

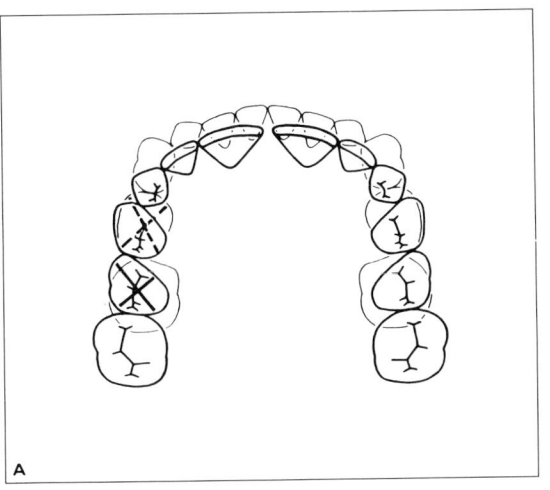
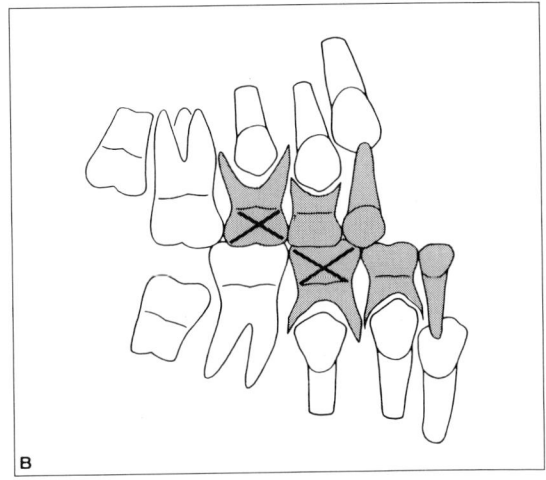
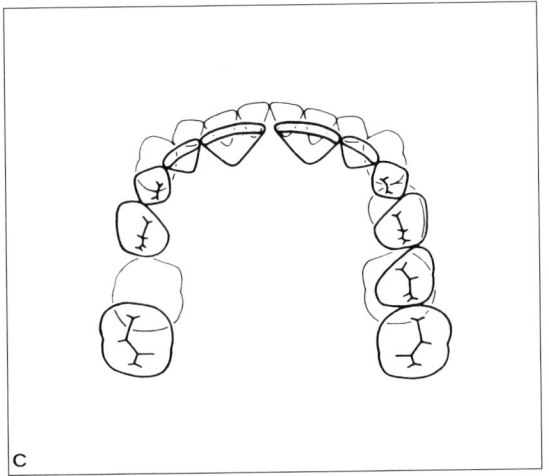
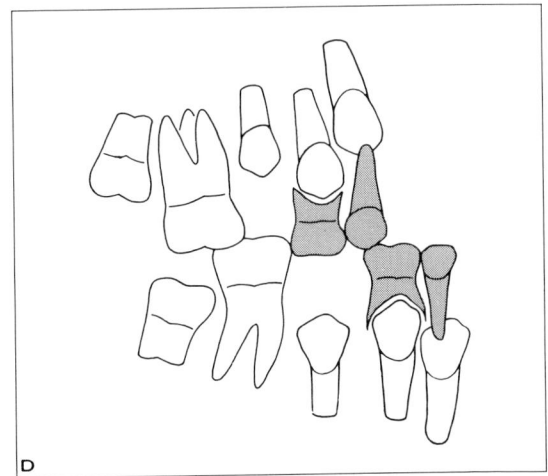

Fig. 15-12 Premature loss of mandibular and maxillary right second deciduous molars in a Class III malocclusion.

A,B The typical occlusal relations allow for overeruption of the maxillary first deciduous molar.
C,D The mesial migration of the mandibular first permanent molar is blocked by the maxillary first deciduous molar in supraposition. The maxillary first permanent molar migrates and rotates mesially.

Results of Premature Loss of Deciduous Teeth

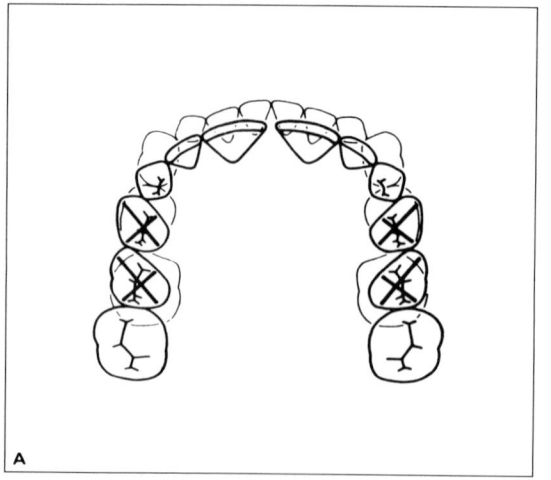
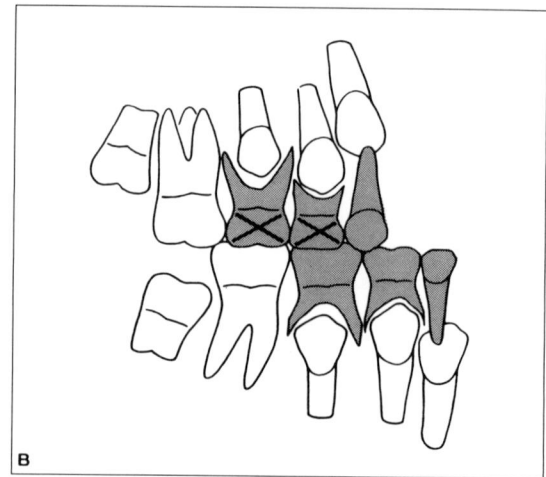
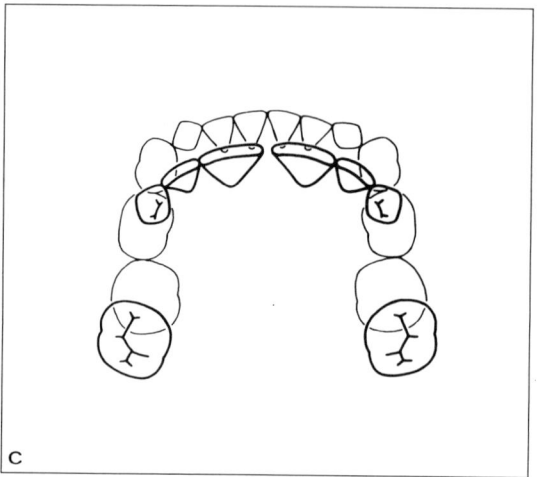
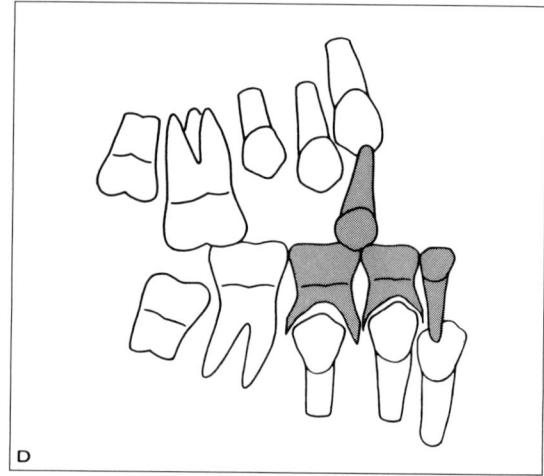

Fig. 15-13 Bilateral premature loss of the maxillary first and second deciduous molars in a Class III malocclusion.

A,B Here too, no overeruption of mandibular deciduous molars can occur.
C,D The maxillary first permanent molars migrate and rotate mesially. The anterior cross bite permits the palatal movement of the maxillary incisors. Accordingly, the reduction in space can be attained in part by distal migration of the mesially positioned teeth.

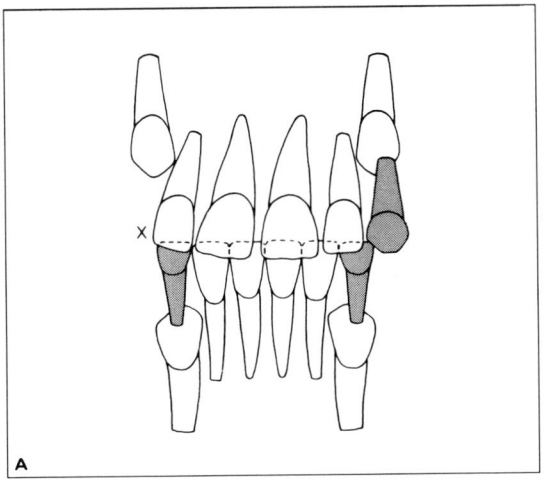
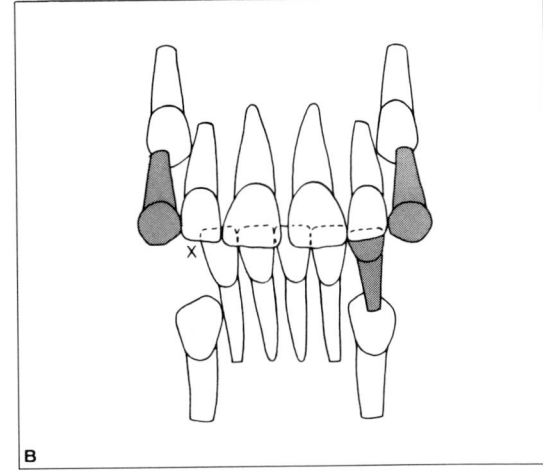
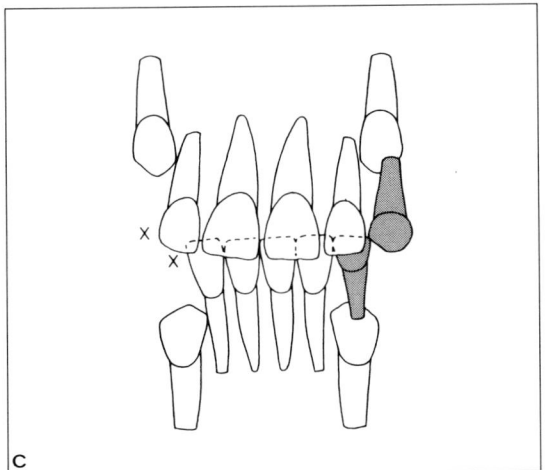
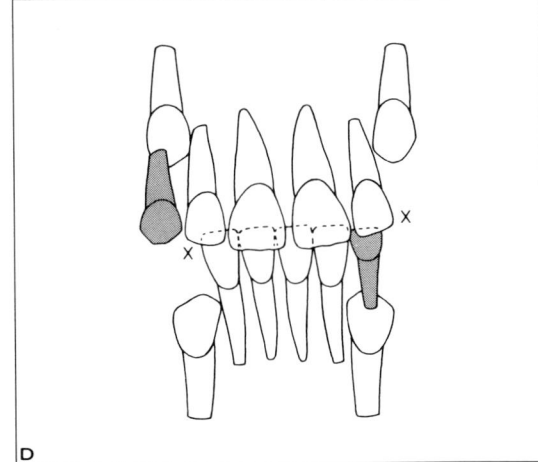

Fig. 15-14 Effects of premature loss of deciduous canines on the angulation of the incisors and on the position of the midpoints of the mandibular and maxillary dental arches.

A Unilateral loss of a maxillary deciduous canine leads to tipping of the maxillary incisors and a deviation of the midpoint of the maxillary dental arch.
B The same is true in the mandible.
C Unilateral loss of the mandibular and maxillary deciduous canines results in tipping of the mandibular and maxillary incisors in the same directions. The midpoints of the two dental arches may still match, but usually do not.
D Loss of one mandibular and one maxillary deciduous canine on different sides. The mandibular and maxillary incisors tip in opposite directions.

largest for the incisor closest to the diastema. In this migration movement, the mesial corner of a maxillary permanent central incisor may cross the median plane (Fig. 15-14A). A corresponding situation may be encountered in the mandible after unilateral premature loss of a deciduous canine (Fig. 15-14B). Unilateral loss of both mandibular and maxillary deciduous canines results in tipping of the maxillary and mandibular incisors in the same direction. The midpoints of the mandibular and maxillary dental arch may still coincide (Fig. 15-14C). After premature loss of a maxillary deciduous canine on one side and a mandibular one on the other, the mandibular and maxillary incisors will tip in opposite directions, with a deviation between the midpoints of the two dental arches accordingly (Fig. 15-14D).

Premature loss of one or two mandibular deciduous molars on one side, or two on one side and one on the other side as a rule results in a midline deviation and in an increase of the overjet and overbite (Fig. 15-15). Bilateral symmetrical loss of one or two mandibular deciduous molars does not lead to midline deviations but usually results in an increase of the overjet and overbite, particularly in a Class II/1 malocclusion (Fig. 15-16). In a Class III malocclusion with an anterior cross bite, premature loss of the maxillary deciduous molars may also result in an increase of the overbite and the reversed overjet (Fig. 15-17).

Results of Premature Loss of Deciduous Teeth

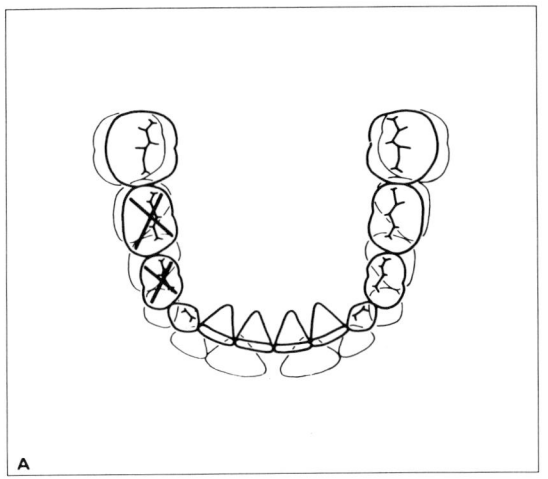
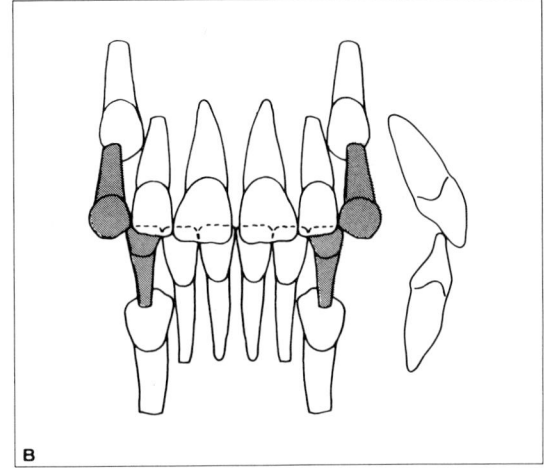
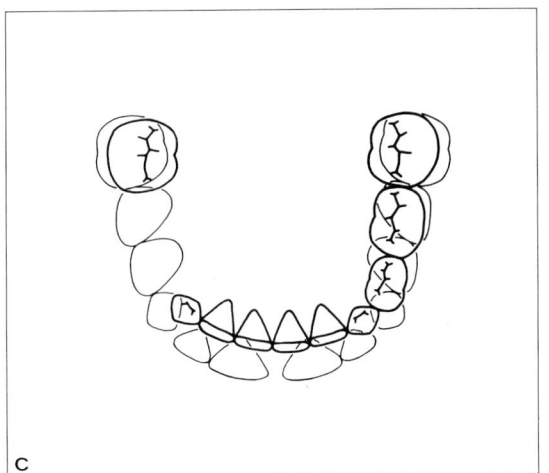
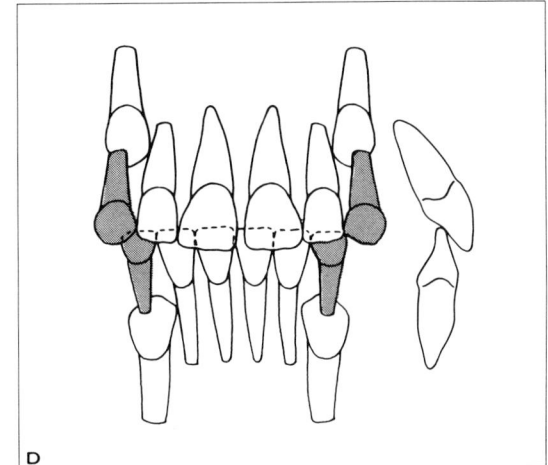

Fig. 15-15 Schematic presentation of the effect of unilateral premature loss of deciduous molars on the overjet and overbite and on the relation of the midpoints of the two dental arches.

A,B Premature loss of the mandibular right first and second deciduous molars in an otherwise normal situation.

C,D The mandibular incisors have tipped to the right side; the midpoints of the two dental arches deviate. The overjet and overbite have increased.

Results of Premature Loss of Deciduous Teeth

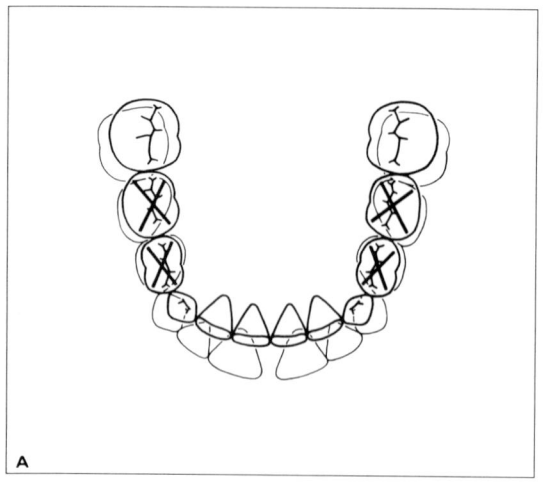
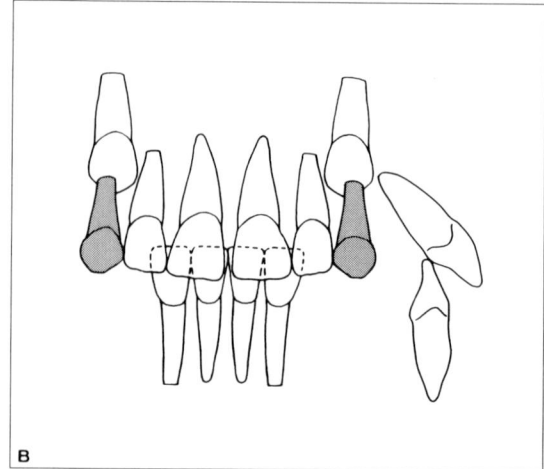
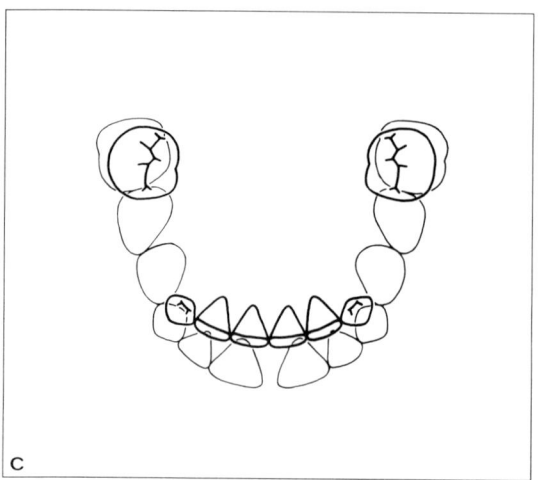
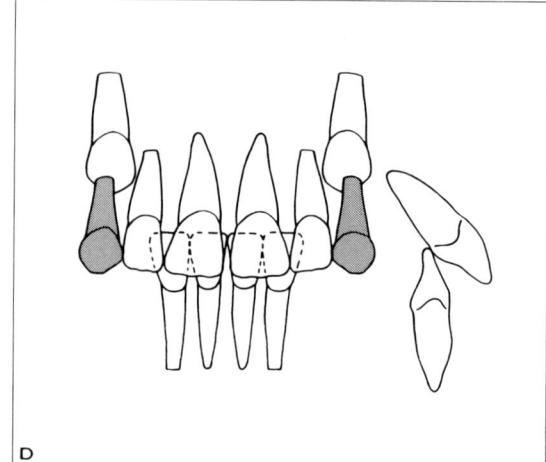

Fig. 15-16 Schematic presentation of the effect of symmetrical loss of mandibular deciduous molars on the overjet and overbite in a Class II/1 malocclusion.

A,B Large overjet and overbite already present prior to the premature loss.
C,D The overjet and overbite have increased.

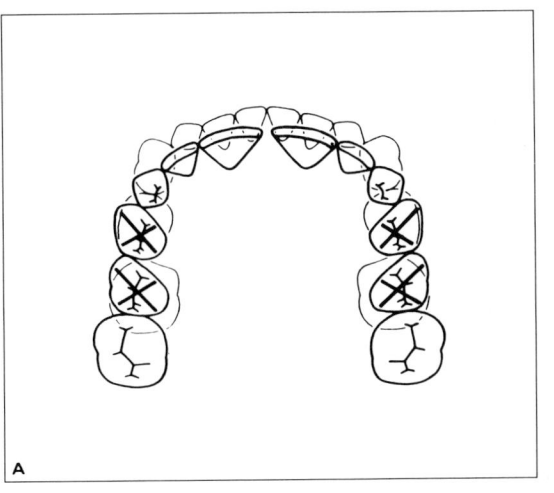 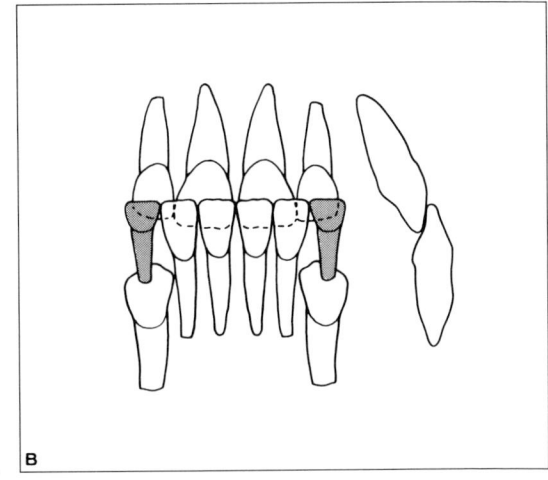
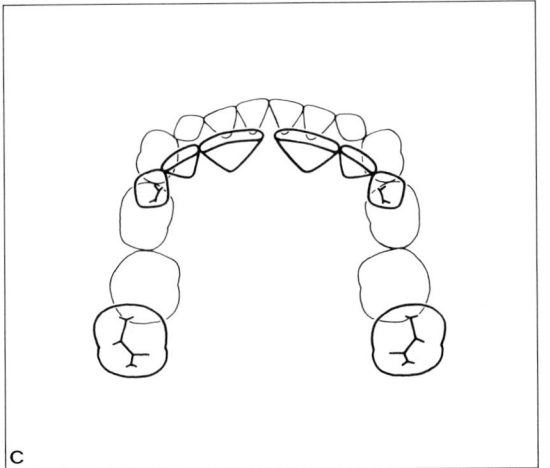 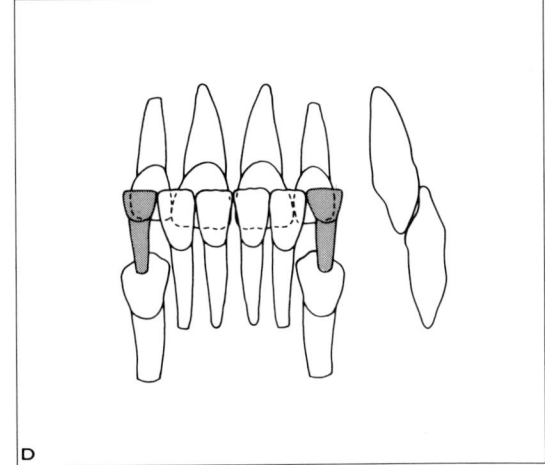

Fig. 15-17 Schematic presentation of the effect of symmetrical loss of maxillary deciduous molars on the overjet and overbite in a Class III malocclusion.

A,B Situation at the time of premature loss.
C,D The overbite and reversed overjet have increased.

Results of Premature Loss of Deciduous Teeth

Table 15-1 describes effects of premature loss of second deciduous molars. Determinants include crowding/spacing, local occlusal relations, jaw relation (Angle), relation of lips to maxillary and mandibular incisors, size of leeway space, and timing of premature loss. Most of the aspects discussed above are represented by abbreviated terms. In addition, the effect of premature loss of second deciduous molars is indicated for different situations.

Table 15-1 Effect of premature loss of second deciduous molars on the space available for their successors

Loss	Class I spacing	Class I crowding	Class II spacing	Class II crowding	Class II lower lip behind maxillary incisors	Class III spacing	Class III crowding
E maxillary	(+)	++	(+)	++	+	(+)	+++
E mandibular		+	(+)	++	+++		(+)
E maxillary and mandibular	(+)	+++	(+)	+++	+++	(+)	++

(+) Space for successor hardly or not at all restricted.
 + Space for successor slightly restricted.
++ Space for successor considerably restricted.
+++ Space for successor very restricted.

Loss of maxillary E: always migration maxillary 6; seldom and limited remigration maxillary 6.

Loss of mandibular E: almost always migration mandibular 6, although often limited; amount of migration mandibular 6 dependent on overeruption of maxillary E and on contact of mandibular 6 with maxillary E; often partial remigration mandibular 6; often no permanent undesirable effect.

Additional factors: midline deviations; increase of overjet; increase of overbite.

Chapter 16

Factors Influencing the Development of the Dentition

The development of the dentition is closely associated with the morphology and growth of the face and the way in which the functions of the orofacial region are exercised.
Purposely, the morphology and growth of the face have been omitted as much as was reasonably possible here.* However, without further explanation it will be clear that the size of the two jaws, their anteroposterior relation, the vertical dimensions of the mandible and the maxilla, as well as the changes occuring during growth in these components play an essential role in the development of the dentition.
The functions of the orofacial region can be classified as those exclusively related to the dentition and face (chewing and partial shaping of the facial configuration) and as those that have a broader character, as respiration, speech and deglutition. Chewing, shaping of the face, and speech will not be discussed here. A few remarks will be made regarding respiration and deglutition.
A restricted passage of the nose usually involves continuous mouth breathing or alternate periods of nose and mouth breathing. However, mouth breathing also can be based on an abnormal habit, while nasal passage is adequate. To attain a good functional relation between the tongue and the lips and cheeks, a closed mouth is a first prerequisite. In non-closed mouth situations, not only the lip seal is lacking, but the tongue and lips cannot fulfill the role that they have to play in maintaining a good relation between the individual teeth, particularly in the incisor region. In the review of open bites (Chapter 13), the effects of abnormal tongue position were discussed. Some comments are made here regarding the role that the tongue and lips have to play in maintaining the position of the mandibular and maxillary incisors.
The position of the incisors is not only determined by the mutual contacts between the pertinent mandibular and maxillary teeth. The tongue and lips have a special function in this respect, as explained in Figures 16.1 and 16.2, together with the

*For this subject, see van der Linden, F.P.G.M. *Facial Growth and Facial Orthopedics.* Quintessence Publ. Co., Chicago, (in press).

Factors Influencing the Development of the Dentition

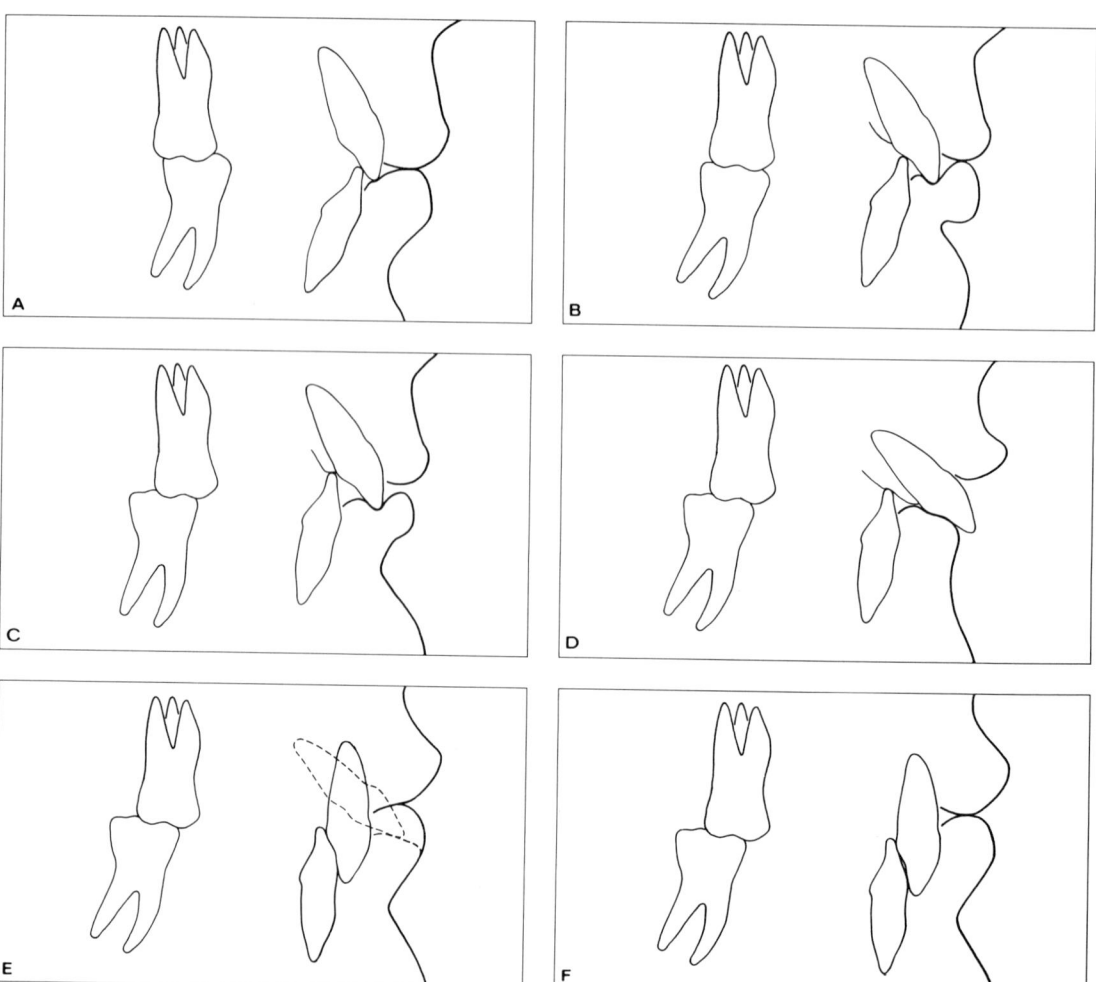

Figure 16-1

Fig. 16-1 Variations in the vertical and sagittal support of the maxillary permanent incisors in normal and abnormal situations.

A   In a Class I condition and normal sagittal and vertical relation in the anterior region, the maxillary incisors are supported vertically by the mandibular incisors on the lingual side and by the lower lip on the labial side. Further, the lower lip also lies against part of the labial surface of the maxillary incisors. The middle of the lipline (stomion) is situated about 1—3 mm superiorly to the incisal edge of the maxillary central incisors. The upper lip exerts a function in preventing the labial displacement of the maxillary incisors. The lower lip also plays a role in this respect, albeit a less important one.

B   In a Class II/1 malocclusion of one-half premolar crown width, the mandibular incisors and often the maxillary ones will also be overerupted. The maxillary incisor is vertically supported by the mandibular incisors, which contact the crowns of the maxillary incisors more cervically than normal. The lower lip provides an essential vertical support for the maxillary incisors.

C   In a more severe Class II/1 malocclusion e.g., of almost one full premolar crown width, the maxillary incisor is not vertically supported by the mandibular incisors, but by the lower lip. The lingually directed force of the lower lip on the maxillary incisor is of little or no importance.

D   In a Class II/1 malocclusion with an extreme overjet, as is often encountered in youngsters with a Class II deviation of one full premolar crown width, the lower lip usually will be positioned behind the maxillary incisors. The mandibular incisors do not contact the palatal surfaces of the maxillary incisors. The lower lip does not lay against the incisal edges of the maxillary incisors. The contact of the lower lip with the palatal surfaces of the maxillary incisors provides only a limited vertical support for the latter. Consequently, the maxillary incisors will erupt further and tip more labially. The position of the lower lip behind the maxillary incisors will lead to an excessive lingual force on the mandibular incisors, which subsequently will tip more lingually and erupt further.

The process described above may become intensified for the labial movement of the maxillary incisors and the lingual tipping of the mandibular ones by thumb or finger sucking. Overeruption of the mandibular incisors will not occur. However, the risk that the lower lip may become positioned behind the maxillary incisors is greater.

E   In a Class II/2 malocclusion with retrusion of the maxillary central incisors and distinct labioversion of the lateral ones (dotted line in this figure), the lower lip usually will cover the labial surfaces of the maxillary central incisors and contact the palatal surfaces of the lateral ones. The vertical support of the maxillary central incisors by the mandibular incisors and the lower lip is of limited value. Overeruption usually will take place until either dental vertical support or contact with the gingiva labially to the mandibular incisors is established. The maxillary lateral incisors are vertically supported by the lower lip, which is positioned more inferiorly at the lateral than at the central incisor level. The lip line describes a curve in transverse direction: high at the median plane, low at the corners of the mouth.

F   In a Class II/2 malocclusion with all four maxillary incisors tipped palatally, the same applies to the lateral ones as stated above for the central ones (E). Vertical support by the lower lip or the mandibular anterior teeth is almost absent. The lower lip exerts a great lingually directed force on the labial surfaces of the maxillary incisors and is responsible for the marked lingual inclination of the maxillary and secondarily also for that of the mandibular incisors. The upper lip does not play a role, or only a negligible one, in the determination of the position of the maxillary incisors, as it does not touch—or only just—these teeth.

Factors Influencing the Development of the Dentition

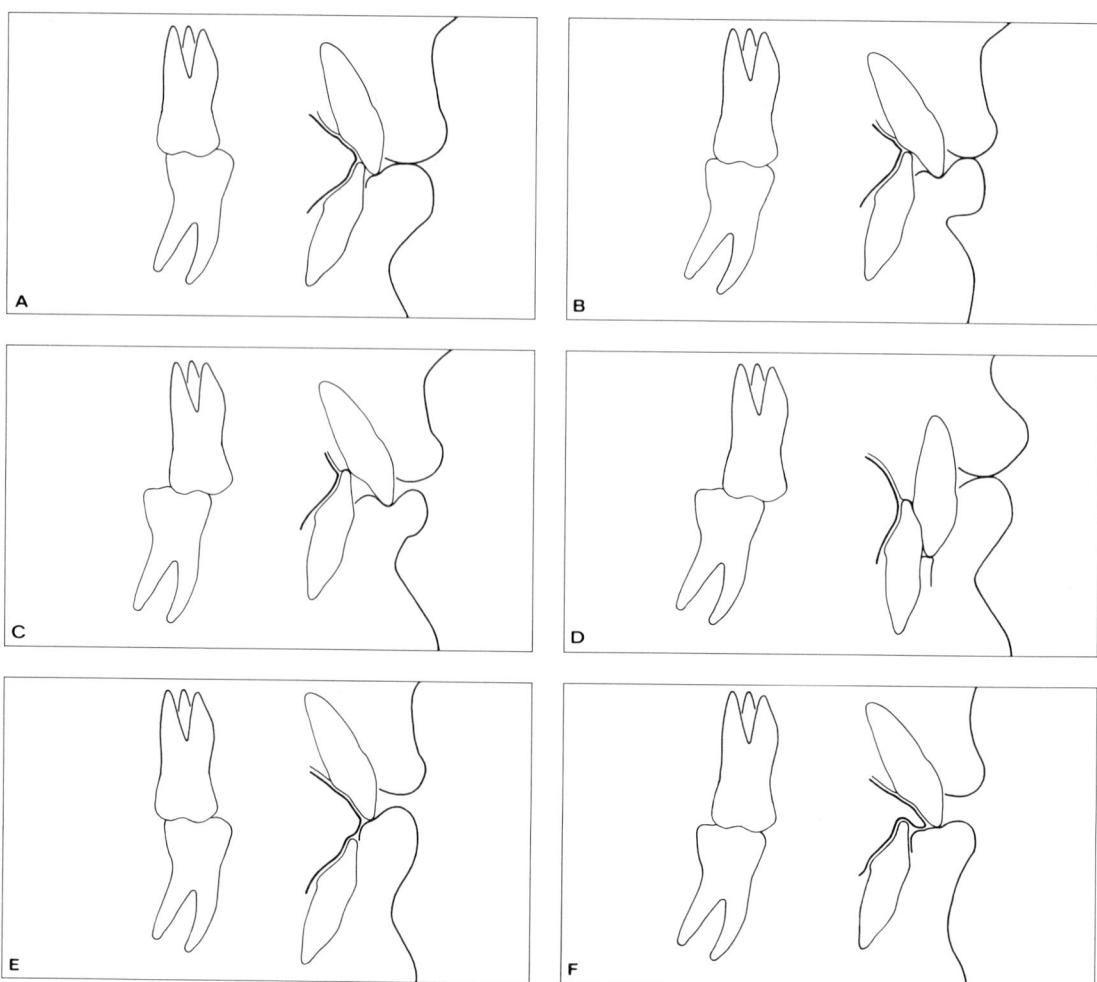

Figure 16-2

Fig. 16-2 Variation in the vertical and sagittal support of the mandibular permanent incisors in normal and abnormal situations.

A   In a Class I condition and normal sagittal and vertical relations in the anterior region, the mandibular incisors are supported vertically by the palatal surfaces of the maxillary incisors. A certain role in this respect may be ascribed to the tongue. Important for the maintenance of the position of the mandibular incisors is the absence of diastemata and the presence of adequate contact points in the mandibular dental arch. The mandibular dental arch provides mutual support for adjacent teeth by good contact points with the mechanical support against buccal forces according to the concept of the design of the Roman arch. In normal situations, the influence exerted by the lower lip on the mandibular incisors is limited regarding the labial support of the mandibular anterior region.

B   In a Class II/1 malocclusion of one-half premolar crown width, the mandibular incisors usually contact the cervical third of the palatal surfaces of the maxillary incisors. The tongue plays the same role in the vertical and lingual support as described above (A).

C   In a more severe Class II/1 malocclusion and a large overjet, the mandibular incisors will not contact the maxillary incisors by erupt until the palate is firmly reached. The tongue is of importance in the sagittal support from the lingual side, together with a possibly existing continuity of the mandibular dental arch. The lower lip plays a role in the support from the labial side.

D   In a Class II/2 malocclusion, the contact between the lingually tipped mandibular and maxillary incisors is usually such that a vertical dental support of the mandibular incisors does not, or almost not, exist. In general, the mandibular incisors erupt until the palate is firmly reached. The influence of the lower lip on the anteroposterior positon of the mandibular incisors is transmitted by the palatally tipped maxillary incisors and exceeds the effect of the counterpressure supplied by the tongue and the supporting features of a continuous mandibular dental arch on the lingual side.

E   In a Class I malocclusion with an open bite, the eruption of the mandibular incisors can be slowed and stopped either by positioning of the tongue over the mandibular incisors or by thumb or finger sucking, or by a combination of both factors. The tongue and lower lip play a role in the anteroposterior positioning of the mandibular incisors. A corresponding situation exists for the maxillary incisors, the tongue, and the upper lip. Furthermore, the lower lip together with the tongue often also play a role in the vertical support of the maxillary incisors.

F   In a Class II/1 malocclusion with an open bite, the mandibular incisors had not erupted until contact was established with the palatal surfaces of the maxillary incisors or the palate. One or more factors have slowed down and stopped the eruption. Also, in such a case, an abnormal tongue position, a thumb or finger sucking habit, or a combination of these are usually causative. The sagittal position of the mandibular incisors depends on the contact between them, and the tongue and the lower lip. In addition, the activity pattern of the lower lip on the one side and the influence of the tongue on the other are essential. The continuity of the mandibular arch is also of importance in this respect. A sagittal and vertical open bite may also be combined with a position of the lower lip partially or totally behind the maxillary incisors, as illustrated in Figure 16-1D. The sagittal position of the maxillary incisors depends on the influence of the tongue on the one side and the upper lip on the other. The lower lip hardly plays a role in this respect, in contrast with the vertical support of the maxillary incisors.

relevancy of the dental contacts. The tongue and the buccal musculature not only play a role in the position of the teeth in the incisor region, they are also of importance in the determination and maintenance of the position and buccolingual inclination of the posterior teeth. In comparison with the anterior region, the influence of the tongue and buccal musculature is relatively small for the posterior teeth, where the intercuspation of the premolars and molars and particularly the transverse interdigitation are more essential in this respect.

Thumb and finger sucking have already been discussed as external factors that influence development of the dentition (Chapters 10 and 13). Also, traumata and premature loss of deciduous teeth, treated in the previous chapter, deserve to be mentioned again in this context.

Chapter 17

Numerical and Graphical Information Concerning Development of the Dentition

The information presented here is based mainly on data derived from investigations carried out in different countries of the western world on the Caucasian race. The information presented includes the following:
—formation and emergence of teeth
—initiation of calcification
—formation stages
—crown dimensions
—eruption speed
—emergence sequences
—occurrence of agenesis of teeth
—various jaw relations

In most instances, the type and the size of the material on which the investigation is based are incorporated in the tables. Occasionally, this information is supplied additionally.

The numerical and graphical information supplied here about different aspects of the development of the dentition forms a selection from a vast amount of data available in the literature. The selection was based mainly on the criterion of providing information that could support different aspects treated in the text. Another purpose was to present in a compact and easily retrievable way some data for which there is no sense in committing.

Dental Arch Dimensions

The data on transverse dental arch dimensions (Tables 17-9 through 17-12) and times of emergence of permanent teeth (Table 17-4) are based on material of the Nymegen Growth Study.[81] A total of 486 boys and girls participated in this study and were followed longitudinally during a 5-year period. The ages were chosen to arrive at overlapping cohorts: from 4 to 9, from 7 to 12, and from 9 to 14 years of age. Every half year, the children were observed and data and material such as impressions of the dental arches were collected. The sample was representative for the population

Table 17-1 Formation of teeth

6th week p.c.*	formation of the dental lamina
8th – 12th week p.c.	I, II, III, IV, V**
4th month p.c.	6**
5th – 6th month p.c.	1, 2, 3
9th month p.c.	4
9th month p.n.*	5, 7
4th year	8 (large variation)

Derived from Stöckli, P.W. Postnataler Wachstumsverlauf, Kieferwachstum und Entwicklung der Dentition. In *Zahnmedizin bei Kindern und Jugendlichen,* ed. R.P. Hotz. Stuttgart: George Thieme Verlag, 1976.
Source: The data in Tables 17-1 and 17-2 are derived from Meyer, W., *Lehrbuch der normalen Histologie und Entwicklungsgeschichte der Zähne des Menschen.* München: J.F. Lehrmanns Verlag, 1932; Broadbent, B.H. *Angle Orthod.* 11(1941):223; Logan, W.H.G., and Kronfeld, R. *J.Amer.Dent.Assn.* 20(1933):379; Moorrees, C.F.A.; Fanning, E.A.; and Hunt, Jr., E.E. *J.Dent.Res.* 42(1963):1490, and Nolla, C.M. *J.Dent.Child.* 27(1960):254.
*p.c.= *postconceptionem:* after conception; p.n. = *postnatal:* after birth
**Roman numerals apply to deciduous teeth; Arabic numerals to permanent teeth.

Table 17-2 Initiation of calcification

5th month p.c.*	I, II**
6th month p.c.	IV, III
7th month p.c.	V
9th month p.c.	6**
6th month p.n.*	−1, +1, −2
12 months	3
18 months	+2
2.5 years	4
3 years	5
3.5 years	7
10 years	8 (large variation)

Derived from Stöckli, see Table 17-1.
Source: See Table 17-1.
*p.c. = *postconceptionem:* after conception; p.n. = *postnatal:* after birth.
**Roman numerals apply to deciduous teeth; Arabic numerals to permanent teeth.
+ = in the maxilla; − = in the mandible.

Table 17-3 Times of emergence of deciduous teeth

6 – 8 months	–I
9 – 10 months	+I
10 – 14 months	II
14 – 18 months	IV
18 – 24 months	III
24 – 30 months	V

Derived from Stöckli, P.W. Postnataler Wachstumsverlauf, Kieferwachstum und Entwicklung der Dentition. In *Zahnmedizin bei Kindern und Jugendlichen,* ed. R.P. Hotz. Stuttgart: George Thieme Verlag, 1976.
Source: Lysell, L.; Magnusson, B.; and Thilander, B. *Odont. Revy* 13(1962):217; Robinow, M.; Richards, T.W.; and Anderson, M. *Growth* 6(1942):127.
+ = in the maxilla; – = in the mandible.

Table 17-4 Calculated emergence times of permanent teeth

Age	Boys			Girls		
	Mean	SD	N	Mean	SD	N
Upper jaw						
1	7.20	.80	166	6.94	.73	224
2	8.22	.88	166	7.97	.96	222
3	11.16	1.68	172	10.89	1.16	250
4	10.27	1.38	172	10.20	1.32	250
5	10.96	1.36	172	10.88	1.52	249
6	6.06	.92	161	6.10	.64	210
7	11.87	1.08	172	11.35	2.22	250
Lower jaw						
1	6.21	.72	166	6.13	.64	221
2	7.36	.73	166	7.21	.75	224
3	10.34	1.05	172	9.56	.98	250
4	10.55	1.73	172	10.09	1.38	250
5	11.44	1.87	172	11.35	1.77	247
6	6.21	.68	166	6.10	.60	215
7	11.31	1.79	172	11.13	1.97	250

Derived from van der Linden, F.P.G.M.; Boersma, H.; and Prahl-Andersen, B. Development of the dentition. In *A mixed-longitudinal interdisciplinary study of growth and development,* eds. B. Prahl-Andersen, C.J. Kowalski, P.H.J. Heydendael. New York: Academic Press, 1979.

Numerical and Graphical Information

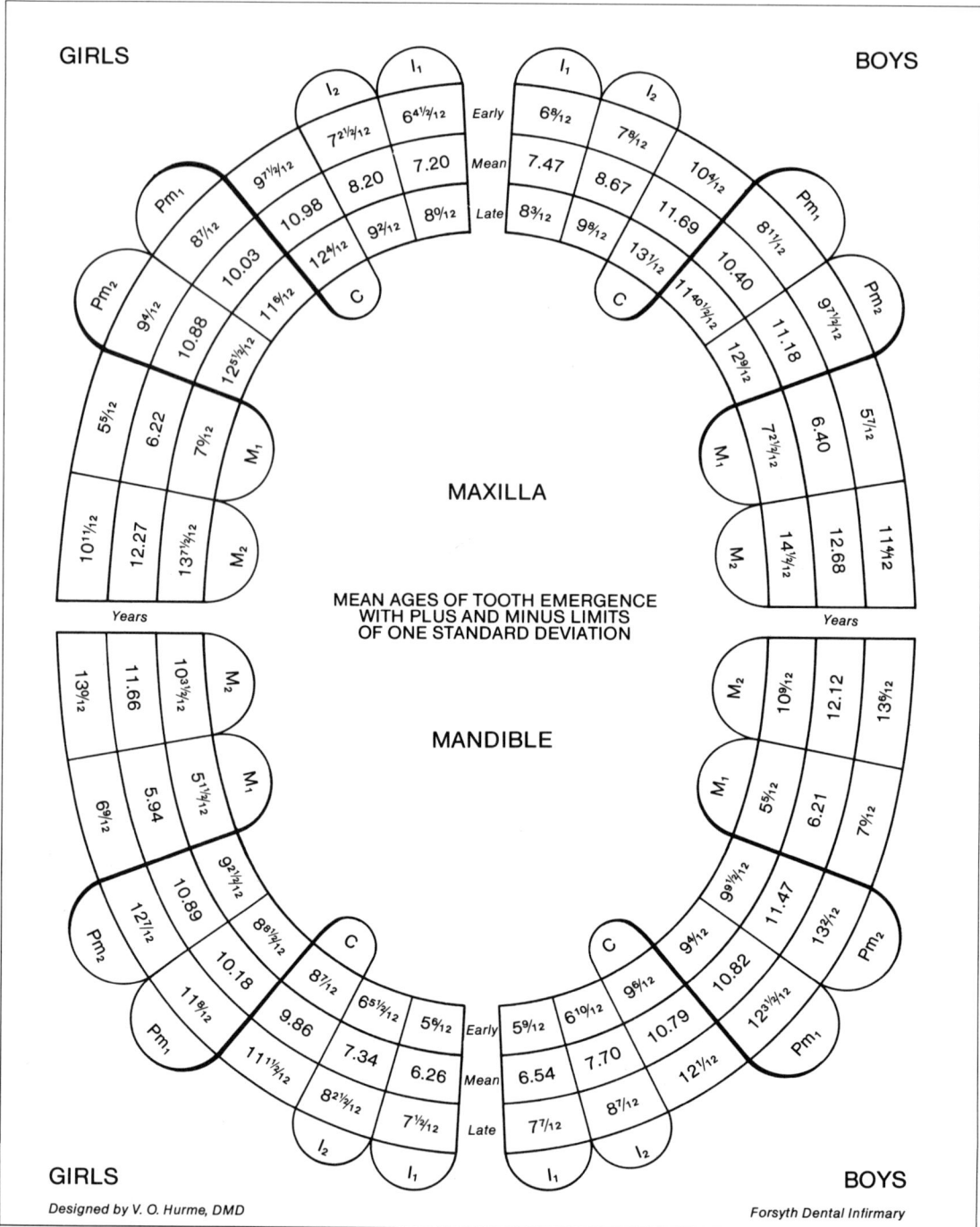

Fig. 17-1 Graphic illustration of early, mean, and late eruption ages for girls (left) and boys (right). Such an age range as depicted would include two-thirds of any sample. (Derived from Hurme, V.O. Ranges of normalcy in the eruption of permanent teeth. J. Dent. Child. 16(1949):11).

of Nymegen and included 25% Class II malocclusions. Because a large part of the sample exhibited orthodontic abnormalities, the data presented here are limited to transverse width dimensions. For more detailed information derived from the Nymegen Growth Study, and particularly regarding the transition of the anterior and posterior teeth, refer to the literature.[4-6,81,104,105,110,112-114]

The data regarding certain changes in the intercanine distance (Tables 17-13 and 17-14), molar occlusion (Table 17-15), and overjet and overbite (Tables 17-16 and 17-17) are based on material from the University School Growth Study of The University of Michigan.[72] In this sample, few and only mild malocclusions are included. Furthermore, these data are not only analyzed on a chronological scale, but also on the basis of biological developmental criteria. An advantage of the latter approach is that derivative values can be plotted against time scales based on certain characteristics of the development of the dentition. This approach has been introduced by Moorrees[64] in the study of the development of the dentition. Some illustrations incorporated in this chapter (Figures 17-6 through 17-9) are derived from his classic work: *The Dentition of the Growing Child.*[63] These illustrations clearly demonstrate the large variation in the changes of the intercanine distances. Not all dental arches become wider at the canine region during the transition of the incisors. This observation is in accordance with the large variations that exists in the spatial conditions of the dental arches. The material on which the figures of Moorrees are based also contain, few and only mild malocclusions.

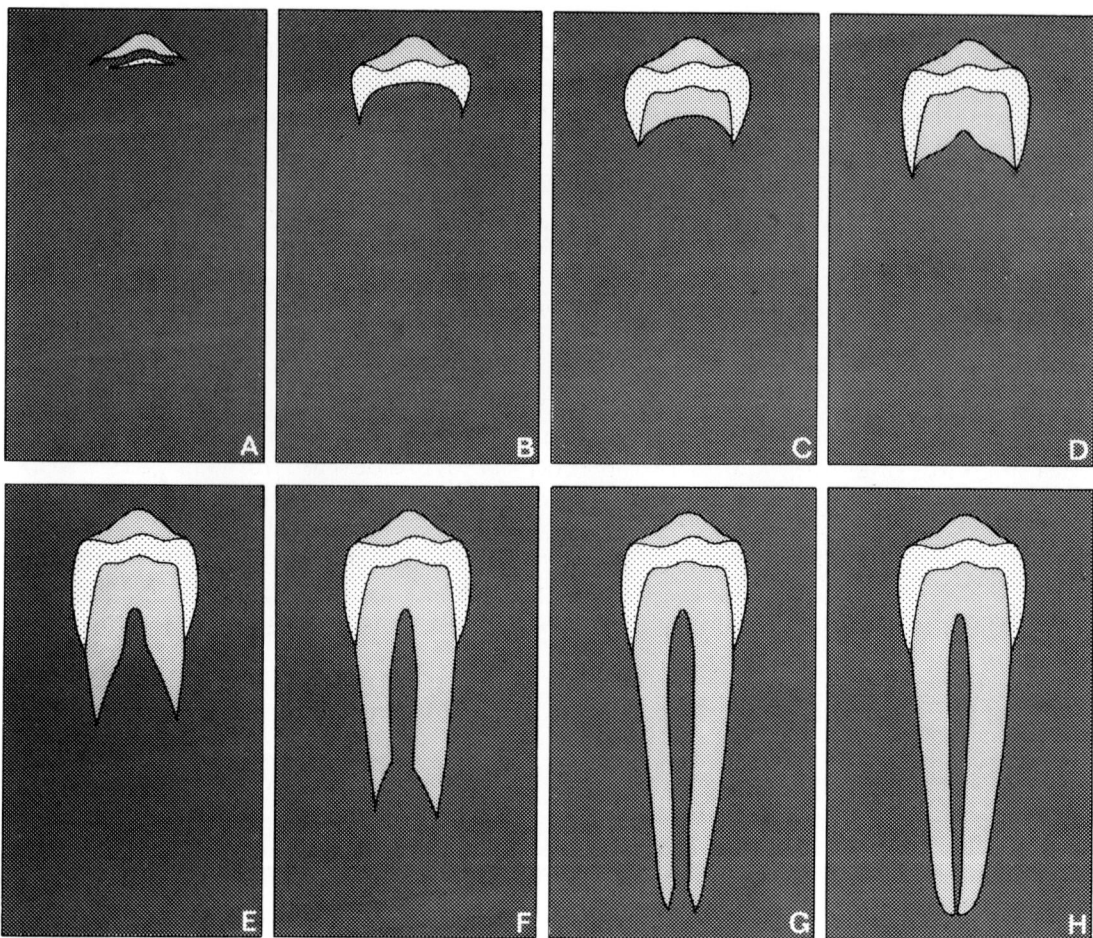

Fig. 17-1 Eight stages of tooth formation of the mandibular first premolar distinguished according to Demerjian et al. 1973.[28] (Figure from Prahl-Andersen, B., and van der Linden, F.P.G.M.[82])

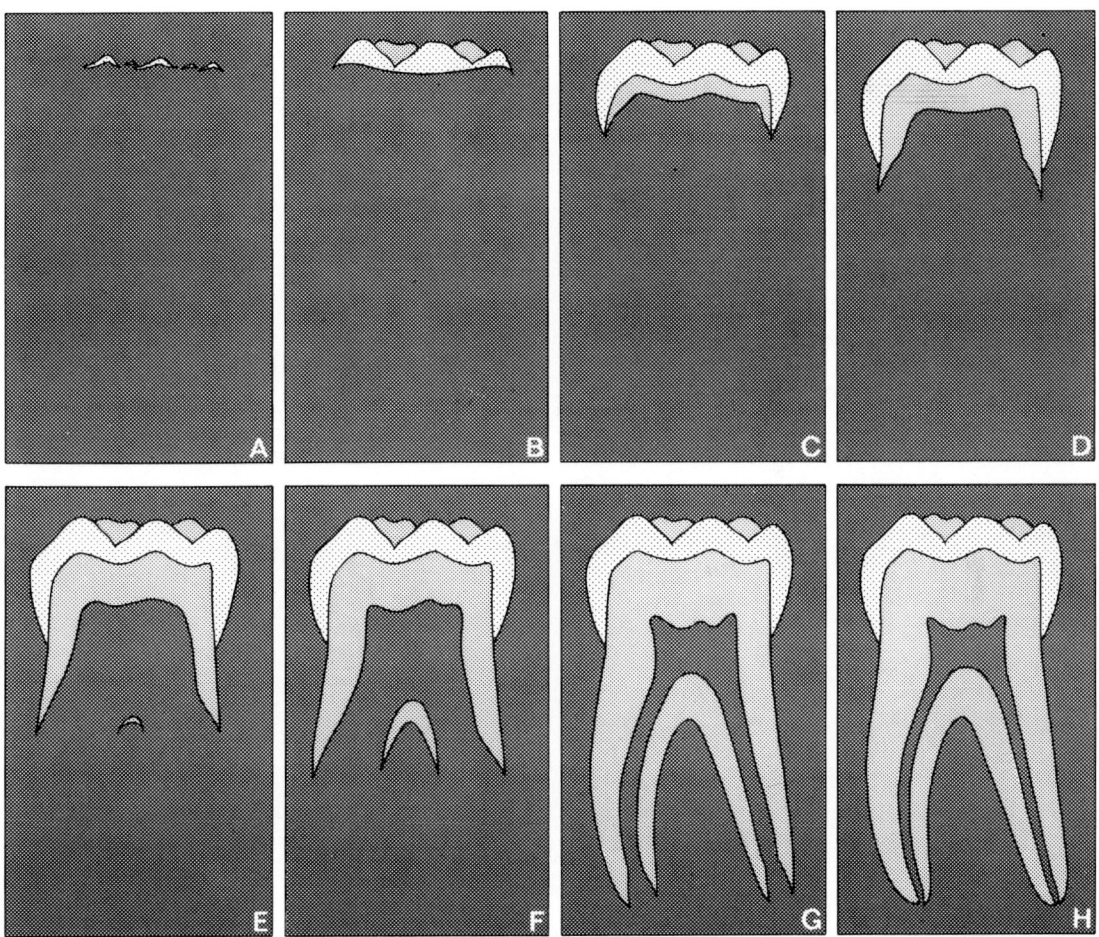

Fig. 17-3 Eight stages of tooth formation of the mandibular first permanent molar, distinguished according to Demerjian et al. 1973.[28] (Figure from Prahl-Andersen, B., and van der Linden, F.P.G.M.[82])

Numerical and Graphical Information

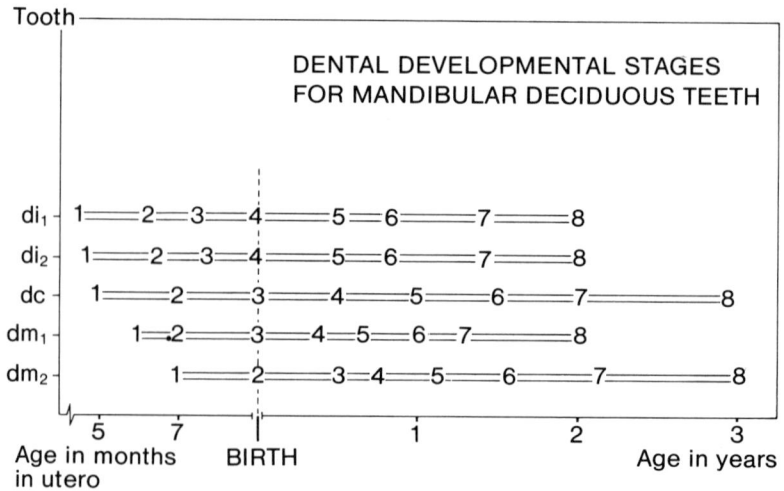

Fig. 17-4 Estimation of the stages of formation of the mandibular deciduous teeth, presented on a time scale. For the stages of formation, refer to Figures 17-2 and 17-3. (Derived from Prahl-Andersen, B., and van der Linden, F.P.G.M.[82])*. di = deciduous tooth e.g., di_1 = mandibular and maxillary central deciduous incisors.

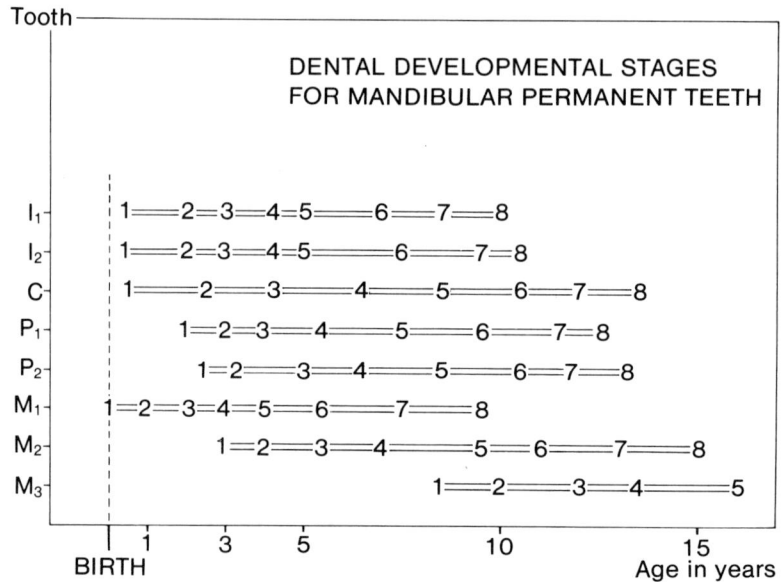

Fig. 17-5 Estimation of the formation stages of the mandibular permanent teeth, presented on a time scale. For the stages of formation, see Figures 17-2 and 17-3. (Derived from Prahl-Andersen, B., and van der Linden, F.P.G.M.[82]).*

*The stages 1 through 8 in Figures 17-4 and 17-5 correspond with the stages A through H in Figures 17-2 and 17-3.

Table 17-5 Mesiodistal crown dimensions

	\multicolumn{3}{c}{Deciduous dentition}				
		Male mean	S.D.		Female mean	S.D.
Tooth	N	mm	mm	N	mm	mm
Maxillary						
central incisor	166	6.41	.43	169	6.48	.43
lateral incisor	189	5.26	.37	175	5.29	.43
canine	212	6.76	.34	194	6.63	.35
first molar	214	6.74	.49	195	6.61	.49
second molar	213	8.84	.53	196	8.74	.47
Mandibular						
central incisor	144	4.06	.35	144	4.10	.31
lateral incisor	182	4.64	.43	171	4.68	.40
canine	213	5.84	.33	193	5.82	.65
first molar	209	7.82	.47	195	7.71	.46
second molar	214	9.90	.52	196	9.73	.48

	\multicolumn{3}{c}{Permanent dentition}				
		Male mean	S.D.		Female mean	S.D.
Tooth	N	mm	mm	N	mm	mm
Maxillary						
central incisor	212	8.91	.59	189	8.67	.57
lateral incisor	201	6.88	.64	172	6.78	.64
canine	152	7.99	.42	125	7.49	.36
first premolar	157	6.76	.47	122	6.60	.46
second premolar	132	6.67	.37	99	6.50	.46
first molar	216	10.58	.56	192	10.18	.58
second molar	121	9.50	.71	80	8.79	.73
Mandibular						
central incisor	214	5.54	.32	196	5.46	.34
lateral incisor	208	6.04	.37	189	5.92	.34
canine	170	6.96	.40	148	6.58	.34
first premolar	159	6.89	.63	134	6.78	.70
second premolar	132	7.22	.47	100	7.07	.46
first molar	215	10.71	.60	191	10.29	.74
second molar	115	9.98	.67	92	9.50	.59

Derived from Moyers, R. E.; van der Linden, F.P.G.M.; Riolo, M.L.; and McNamara, Jr., J.A. *Standards of human occlusal development.* Monograph No. 5., Craniofacial Growth Series. Center for Human Growth and Development. The University of Michigan, Ann Arbor, 1976.

Table 17-6 Correlations in emergence age of permanent mandibular teeth in females

	I_2	C	Pm_1	Pm_2	M_1	M_2
I_1	.85	.78	.64	.43	.59	.44
I_2		.83	.70	.53	.62	.58
C			.78	.59	.56	.58
Pm_1				.65	.55	.58
Pm_2					.48	.64
M_1						.76

Derived from Moorrees, C.F.A., and Kent, R.L. Patterns of dental maturation. In *The biology of occlusal development*, ed. J.A. McNamara, Jr. Monograph No. 7., Craniofacial Growth Series. Center for Human Growth and Development. The University of Michigan, Ann Arbor, 1977.

Table 17-7 Correlation coefficients for mesiodistal crown diameters of deciduous and permanent teeth*

Tooth	I_1	I_2	C	Pm_1	Pm_2	M_1	M_2
Maxilla							
di_1	0.63	0.36	0.35	0.33	0.31	0.40	0.28
di_2	0.32	0.31	0.29	0.27	0.22	0.19	0.25
dc	0.27	0.26	0.29	0.42	0.31	0.25	0.35
dm_1	0.34	0.25	0.35	0.34	0.41	0.36	0.45
dm_2	0.32	0.26	0.23	0.39	0.38	0.51	0.39
Mandible							
di_1	0.43	0.41	0.32	0.24	0.29	0.28	0.26
di_2	0.42	0.44	0.39	0.15	0.24	0.35	0.32
dc	0.30	0.30	0.26	0.25	0.36	0.25	0.34
dm_1	0.29	0.38	0.44	0.47	0.51	0.45	0.42
dm_2	0.24	0.37	0.35	0.39	0.41	0.53	0.43

Derived from Moorrees, C.F.A., and Reeds, R.B. Correlations among crown diameters of human teeth. *Arch. Oral Biol.* 9 (1964): 685.
*The numbers of individuals studied ranged from 121 to 153, except for correlations involving the second permanent second molars ($n = 68–72$).

Table 17-8 Correlation coefficients for the mesiodistal crown diameters of corresponding groups of deciduous and permanent teeth

Tooth groups		Males		Females	
		$r \pm S.E._r$	Number	$r \pm S.E._r$	Number
Maxilla					
di_1+di_2	I_1+I_2........	+0.31±0.11	62	+0.55±0.09	58
$d_c+dm_1+dm_2$	$C+Pm_1+Pm_2$..	+0.45±0.10	62	+0.55±0.09	58
Mandible					
di_1+di_2	I_1+I_2........	+0.39±0.11	58	+0.44±0.10	61
$d_c+dm_1+dm_2$	$C+Pm_1+Pm_2$..	+0.57±0.09	58	+0.59±0.08	61

Derived from Moorrees, C.F.A., and Chadha, J.M. Crown diameters of corresponding tooth groups in the deciduous and permanent dentition. *J.Dent.Res.* 41(1962):466.

Table 17-9

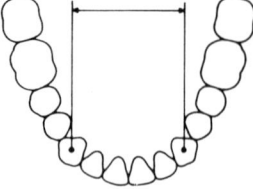

$\overline{3}-\overline{3}$
Arch width: mandibular canines (distance between the mandibular canines at the cusp tips in mm).

Age	Male N	Male Mean	Male SD	Female N	Female Mean	Female SD
4.0	29	23.64	1.46	35	23.19	1.70
4.5	35	23.52	1.34	26	22.81	1.43
5.0	26	23.84	1.65	34	23.39	1.66
5.5	59	23.98	1.69*	59	23.32	1.74
6.0	59	24.11	1.90	59	23.61	1.91
6.5	56	24.73	2.09	57	24.47	2.14
7.0	89	25.31	2.09	105	24.90	2.32
7.5	130	26.07	2.00	130	25.56	2.18
8.0	124	26.52	1.93*	125	25.92	2.06
8.5	120	26.86	2.09**	127	25.97	2.04
9.0	98	26.48	1.70**	97	25.62	1.83
9.5	137	26.32	1.97**	173	25.65	1.87
10.0	135	26.68	1.88**	169	25.68	1.73
10.5	132	26.52	1.91**	167	25.63	1.64
11.0	132	26.43	2.02**	168	25.63	1.74
11.5	133	26.54	1.98**	166	25.65	1.73
12.0	98	26.58	1.97**	121	25.73	1.69
12.5	61	26.10	1.81	88	25.65	1.87
13.0	59	26.11	1.87	83	25.79	1.93
13.5	59	26.17	1.88	83	25.86	1.90
14.0	59	26.35	2.00	83	25.88	1.92

Source: See Table 17-4.
*A single asterisk indicates sexual dimorphism that is significantly different at the 5% level of confidence.
**Double asterisks indicate sexual dimorphism significantly different at the 1% level of confidence.

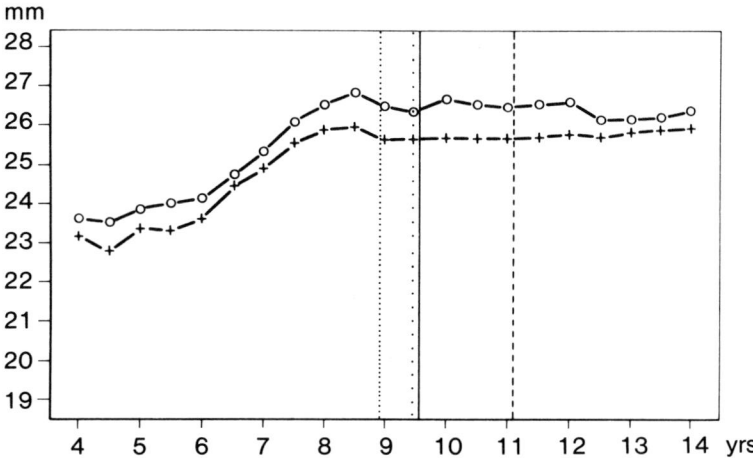

Last appearance of mandibular deciduous canine in girls (.....); in boys(. . . . .). First appearance of mandibular permanent canine in girls (———); in boys (- - - -).

Table 17-10

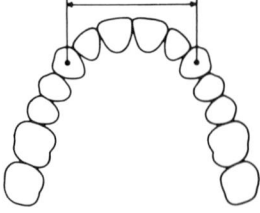

3-3
Arch width: maxillary canines (distance between the maxillary canines at the cusp tips in mm).

Age	N	Male Mean	SD	N	Female Mean	SD
4.0	29	28.71	2.20	35	28.12	1.89
4.5	35	28.80	1.40*	27	27.94	1.42
5.0	26	28.94	2.24	34	28.23	1.87
5.5	59	28.84	1.88*	60	28.03	1.69
6.0	59	28.82	1.94*	59	28.15	1.75
6.5	56	29.63	2.10	58	28.90	1.99
7.0	90	30.26	2.30*	107	29.61	2.10
7.5	131	30.71	2.16*	135	30.07	2.03
8.0	127	31.21	2.11**	130	30.44	2.08
8.5	124	31.42	2.06**	131	30.43	2.10
9.0	100	31.38	1.98**	97	30.16	1.99
9.5	135	31.58	2.02**	157	30.78	2.11
10.0	129	32.20	2.11**	154	31.36	1.95
10.5	121	32.25	2.21**	154	31.43	1.98
11.0	125	32.78	2.36**	158	31.91	2.03
11.5	125	33.17	2.32**	157	32.21	2.37
12.0	93	33.93	2.30**	114	32.67	2.18
12.5	60	34.05	2.13**	83	32.77	2.19
13.0	58	34.26	2.13**	80	33.02	2.39
13.5	59	34.46	2.25**	81	33.08	2.47
14.0	59	34.63	2.11**	82	33.08	2.14

Source: See Table 17-4.
*See Table 17-9.
**See Table 17-9.

Numerical and Graphical Information

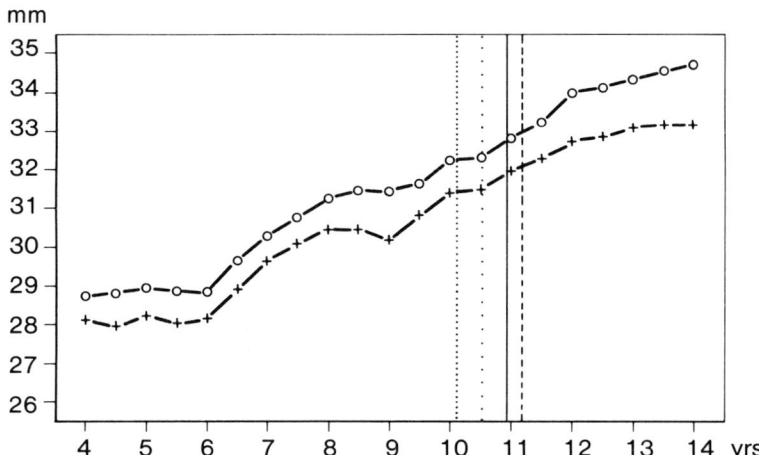

Last appearance of maxillary deciduous canine in girls (·····); in boys (· · · · ·). First appearance of maxillary permanent canine in girls (———); in boys (- - - -).

Table 17-11

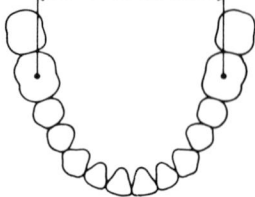

6̄ - 6̄
Arch width: mandibular first molars (distance between the mandibular first molars at the centroids in mm).[a]

Age	N	Male Mean	SD	N	Female Mean	SD
7.0	87	39.94	3.24	107	39.71	3.18
7.5	125	41.16	2.61**	139	40.14	2.37
8.0	124	41.38	2.19**	137	40.37	2.32
8.5	127	41.68	2.32**	138	40.67	2.41
9.0	106	41.49	2.52**	105	40.43	2.24
9.5	146	41.34	2.53**	173	40.26	2.41
10.0	141	41.82	2.61**	169	40.68	2.45
10.5	135	41.85	2.54**	168	40.76	2.45
11.0	133	41.86	2.56**	165	40.83	2.46
11.5	133	41.90	2.78**	163	40.96	2.44
12.0	97	42.41	2.75**	116	41.32	2.44
12.5	58	42.84	2.62**	84	41.60	2.44
13.0	56	42.72	2.44*	79	41.60	2.52
13.5	56	42.66	2.45**	79	41.49	2.39
14.0	56	42.63	2.42**	79	41.43	2.50

Source: See Table 17-4.

[a]The information available on mandibular first molar width prior to 7 years of age is not incorporated in the table and graph.
*See Table 17-9.
**See Table 17-9.

Numerical and Graphical Information

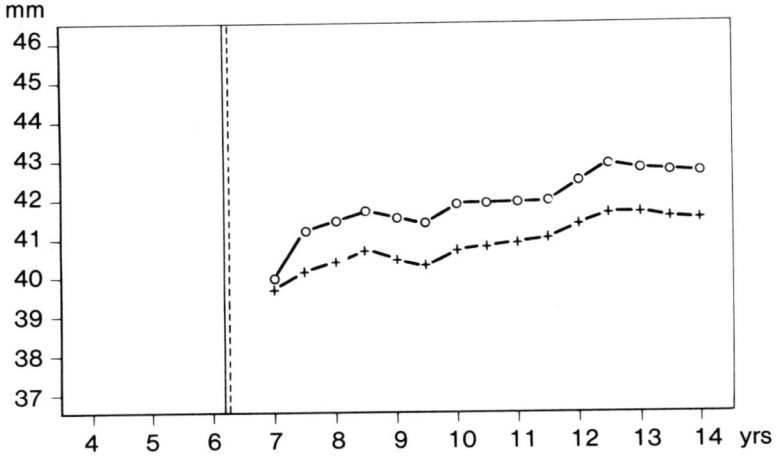

First appearance of mandibular permanent first molar in girls (———); in boys (- - - -).

Table 17-12

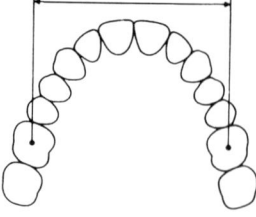

6 - 6
Arch width: maxillary first molars (distance between the maxillary first molars at the centroids in mm).[a]

Age	N	Male Mean	SD	N	Female Mean	SD
7.0	90	42.41	2.56	107	42.32	2.38
7.5	133	43.86	2.59**	138	43.01	2.24
8.0	129	44.41	2.19**	137	43.34	2.29
8.5	128	44.51	2.16**	139	43.43	2.25
9.0	107	44.67	2.24**	104	43.61	2.28
9.5	146	45.15	2.50**	172	43.94	2.32
10.0	140	45.04	2.55**	168	43.90	2.40
10.5	129	45.31	2.57**	160	44.09	2.46
11.0	126	45.39	2.61**	158	44.19	2.43
11.5	125	45.45	2.61**	156	44.29	2.44
12.0	95	45.72	2.47**	111	44.32	2.26
12.5	56	45.59	2.50**	77	44.13	2.10
13.0	54	45.80	2.59**	74	44.28	2.12
13.5	54	45.89	2.56**	75	44.37	2.12
14.0	55	45.87	2.73**	76	44.43	1.96

Source: See Table 17-4.
[a]The information available on maxillary first molar width prior to seven years of age is not incorporated in the table and graph.
**See Table 17-9.

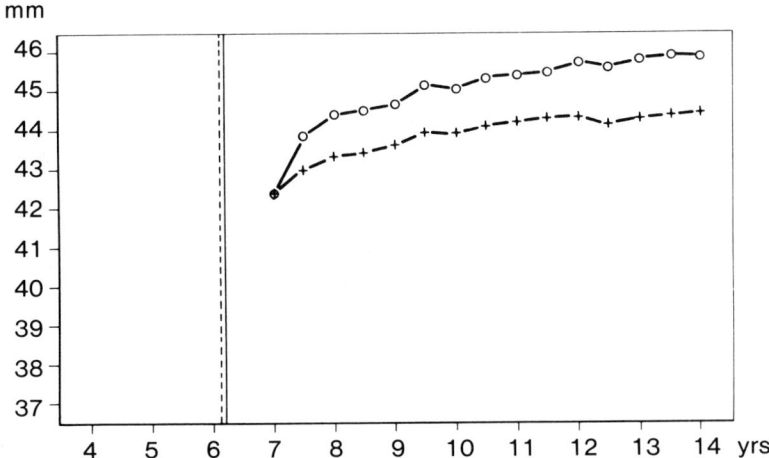

First appearance of maxillary permanent first molar in girls (———); in boys (- - - -).

Table 17-13

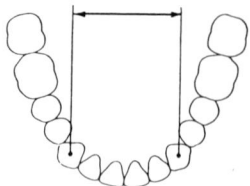

3–3

Arch width: mandibular canines
Developmental age: mandibular central incisor eruption (approx. 6.5 yrs after birth).
Distance between the mandibular canines at the centroids. Age is based on the first appearance of a permanent mandibular central incisor.

		Deciduous						Permanent				
		Male			Female			Male			Female	
Age	N	mean mm	S.D. mm	N	mean mm	S.D. mm	N	mean mm	S.D. mm	N	mean mm	S.D. mm
−9	0	—	—	0	—	—	0	—	—	0	—	—
−8	0	—	—	0	—	—	0	—	—	0	—	—
−7	0	—	—	0	—	—	0	—	—	0	—	—
−6	0	—	—	0	—	—	0	—	—	0	—	—
−5	0	—	—	1	19.40	—	0	—	—	0	—	—
−4	4	22.19	1.16	2	20.83	0.90	0	—	—	0	—	—
−3	20	21.56	1.29	18	21.62	1.13	0	—	—	0	—	—
−2	40	21.62	1.17	39	21.69	1.31	0	—	—	0	—	—
−1	65	21.88	1.40	70	21.64	1.39	0	—	—	0	—	—
0	64	22.99	1.70	69	22.55	1.55	0	—	—	0	—	—
+1	56	24.14	1.93	64	23.60	1.71	0	—	—	0	—	—
+2	47	24.82	1.65*	61	24.07	1.52	0	—	—	0	—	—
+3	39	24.89	1.68	33	24.20	1.24	0	—	—	1	25.10	—
+4	23	24.86	1.67	3	24.75	0.88	1	25.90	—	13	24.53	0.96
+5	5	25.68	0.75	0	—	—	13	25.26	1.25	32	24.57	1.29
+6	0	—	—	0	—	—	27	25.00	1.45	31	24.54	1.26
+7	0	—	—	0	—	—	27	24.80	1.10	26	24.42	1.27
+8	0	—	—	0	—	—	22	24.78	1.25	20	24.12	1.61
+9	0	—	—	0	—	—	21	24.77	1.53	13	23.77	1.80
+10	0	—	—	0	—	—	14	25.04	1.65	11	23.58	1.91

Source: See Table 17-5.
*See Table 17-9.

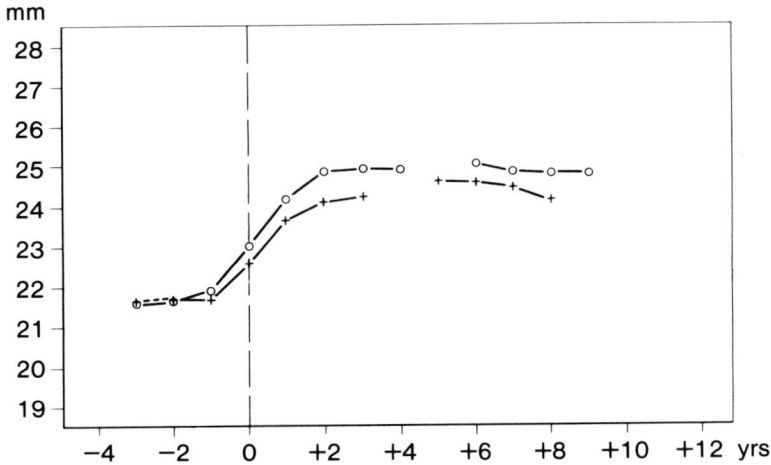

Table 17-14

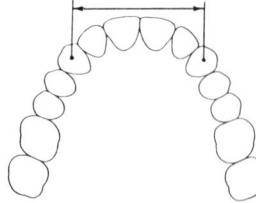

3–3
Arch width: maxillary canines
Developmental age: mandibular central incisor eruption (approx. 6.5 yrs after birth).
Distance between the maxillary canines at the centroids. Age is based on the first appearance of a permanent mandibular central incisor.

	Deciduous						Permanent					
		Male			Female			Male			Female	
Age	N	mean mm	S.D. mm	N	mean mm	S.D. mm	N	mean mm	S.D. mm	N	mean mm	S.D. mm
−9	0	—	—	0	—	—	0	—	—	0	—	—
−8	0	—	—	0	—	—	0	—	—	0	—	—
−7	0	—	—	0	—	—	0	—	—	0	—	—
−6	0	—	—	0	—	—	0	—	—	0	—	—
−5	0	—	—	1	24.60	—	0	—	—	0	—	—
−4	4	26.93	1.55	2	25.82	1.55	0	—	—	0	—	—
−3	21	26.43	1.22	19	26.43	1.49	0	—	—	0	—	—
−2	42	26.99	1.26*	40	26.26	1.44	0	—	—	0	—	—
−1	67	27.14	1.50**	72	26.47	1.49	0	—	—	0	—	—
0	66	27.88	1.64*	71	27.25	1.72	0	—	—	0	—	—
+1	59	29.29	1.92*	65	28.57	1.84	0	—	—	0	—	—
+2	53	30.11	1.87	65	29.43	1.90	0	—	—	0	—	—
+3	52	30.32	1.97*	50	29.48	1.87	0	—	—	0	—	—
+4	40	30.17	1.80	32	29.31	1.86	0	—	—	0	—	—
+5	21	30.41	1.79	7	29.66	2.46	2	32.11	0.15	6	32.66	2.24
+6	0	—	—	0	—	—	13	32.57	1.69*	22	30.99	2.22
+7	0	—	—	0	—	—	23	32.25	1.24*	22	31.29	1.41
+8	0	—	—	0	—	—	21	32.26	1.78	21	31.43	1.40
+9	0	—	—	0	—	—	21	32.38	2.28	13	31.19	1.68
+10	0	—	—	0	—	—	15	32.24	2.37	12	31.12	1.53

Source: See Table 17-5.
*See Table 17-9.
**See Table 17-9.

Numerical and Graphical Information

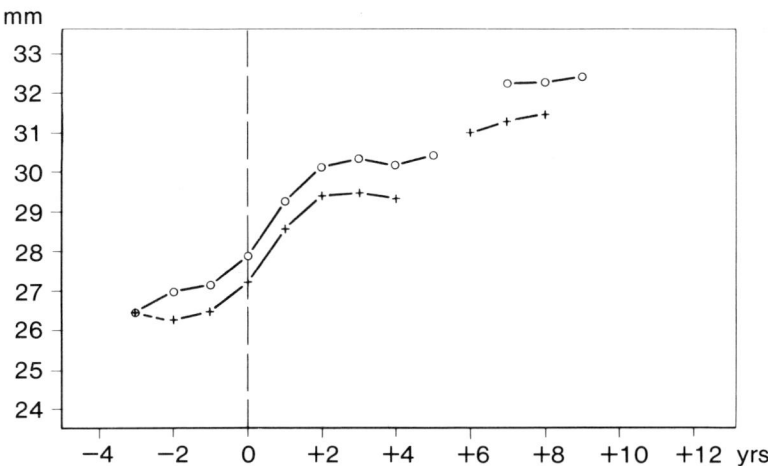

Table 17-15

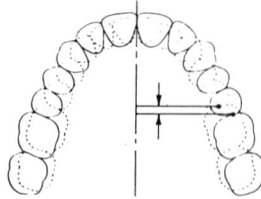

6̲ / 6̄
Anteroposterior occlusal relations: maxillary and mandibular first molars
Developmental age: mandibular central incisor eruption (approx. 6.5 yrs after birth).
Anteroposterior distance between the maxillary and mandibular first molars at the mesial midpoints. Age is based on the first appearance of a permanent mandibular central incisor.

Age	N	Male mean mm	S.D. mm		N	Female mean mm	S.D. mm
-9	0	—	—		0	—	—
-8	0	—	—		0	—	—
-7	0	—	—		0	—	—
-6	0	—	—		0	—	—
-5	0	—	—		0	—	—
-4	0	—	—		0	—	—
-3	0	—	—		0	—	—
-2	0	—	—		0	—	—
-1	1	-6.08	—		0	—	—
0	1	-2.17	—		1	1.60	—
+1	28	0.58	1.59		30	0.51	1.46
+2	51	0.40	1.66	*	61	1.08	1.65
+3	57	0.56	1.55		57	0.99	1.45
+4	51	0.94	1.40		53	1.18	1.61
+5	46	1.24	1.54		44	1.49	1.57
+6	36	1.44	1.17		35	1.84	1.75
+7	28	1.97	1.41		27	1.95	1.24
+8	23	1.94	1.74		22	2.31	1.44
+9	21	1.44	1.98		13	2.49	0.91
+10	15	1.23	2.32	*	12	2.92	1.03

Source: See Table 17-5.
*See Table 17-9.

Numerical and Graphical Information

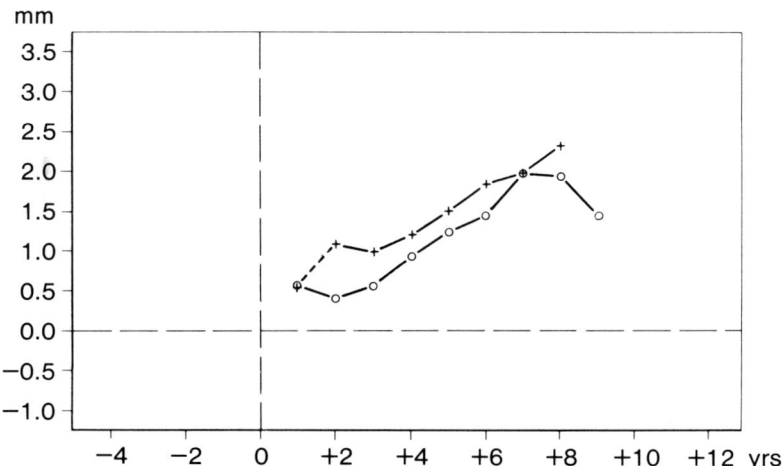

Table 17-16

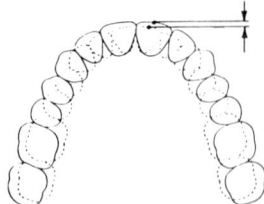

1̲/1̲
Anteroposterior occlusal relations: maxillary and mandibular central incisors.
Developmental age: mandibular central incisor eruption (approx. 6.5 yrs after birth).
Anteroposterior distance between the maxillary and mandibular central incisors at the most labial points. Age is based on the first appearance of a permanent mandibular central incisor.

	Deciduous						Permanent					
		Male mean mm	S.D. mm		Female mean mm	S.D. mm		Male mean mm	S.D. mm		Female mean mm	S.D. mm
Age	N			N			N			N		
−9	0	—	—	0	—	—	0	—	—	0	—	—
−8	0	—	—	0	—	—	0	—	—	0	—	—
−7	0	—	—	0	—	—	0	—	—	0	—	—
−6	0	—	—	0	—	—	0	—	—	0	—	—
−5	0	—	—	1	2.99	—	0	—	—	0	—	—
−4	4	1.73	2.66	1	6.11	—	0	—	—	0	—	—
−3	21	2.63	1.48	19	3.45	1.99	0	—	—	0	—	—
−2	41	2.72	1.47	36	3.49	2.21	0	—	—	0	—	—
−1	56	2.90	1.47	64	3.03	2.07	0	—	—	0	—	—
0	6	2.92	1.76	4	1.66	1.89	0	—	—	0	—	—
+1	0	—	—	0	—	—	8	3.90	1.99	8	3.55	1.84
+2	0	—	—	0	—	—	36	4.08	2.29	45	3.25	2.12
+3	0	—	—	0	—	—	54	4.00	1.94	55	3.69	2.47
+4	0	—	—	0	—	—	49	3.81	1.70	51	3.68	2.16
+5	0	—	—	0	—	—	45	3.64	1.77	41	3.38	1.88
+6	0	—	—	0	—	—	35	4.04	1.60*	34	3.09	1.94
+7	0	—	—	0	—	—	26	3.30	1.19	26	2.94	1.50
+8	0	—	—	0	—	—	21	3.21	1.46	20	3.15	1.04
+9	0	—	—	0	—	—	21	3.16	1.58	12	3.34	1.18
+10	0	—	—	0	—	—	14	3.15	1.21	11	3.32	1.09

Source: See Table 17-5.
*See Table 17-9.

Numerical and Graphical Information

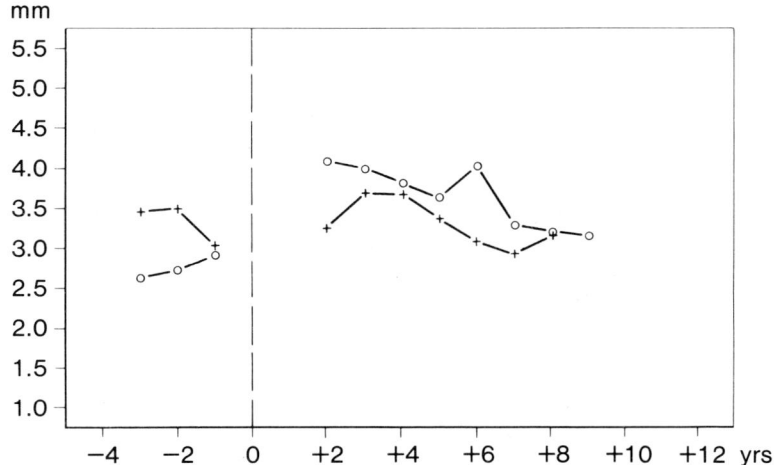

Table 17-17*

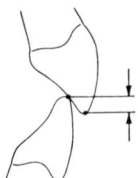

1/ T̄
Vertical occlusal relations: maxillary and mandibular central incisors.
Developmental age: mandibular central incisor eruption (approx. 6.5 yrs after birth).
Vertical distance between the maxillary and mandibular central incisors at the highest points. Age is based on the first appearance of a permanent mandibular central incisor.
(Variable 1347)

| | | Deciduous | | | | | | Permanent | | | |
| | | Male | | | Female | | | Male | | | Female | |
Age	N	mean mm	S.D. mm	N	mean mm	S.D. mm	N	mean mm	S.D. mm	N	mean mm	S.D. mm
-9	0	—	—	0	—	—	0	—	—	0	—	—
-8	0	—	—	0	—	—	0	—	—	0	—	—
-7	0	—	—	0	—	—	0	—	—	0	—	—
-6	0	—	—	0	—	—	0	—	—	0	—	—
-5	0	—	—	1	0.90	—	0	—	—	0	—	—
-4	4	1.40	1.36	2	1.85	3.46	0	—	—	0	—	—
-3	20	1.01	1.68	17	0.54	1.95	0	—	—	0	—	—
-2	39	0.99	1.69	37	0.27	1.72	0	—	—	0	—	—
-1	52	1.16	1.65	61	0.94	1.75	0	—	—	0	—	—
0	6	1.07	2.35	4	0.05	1.38	0	—	—	0	—	—
+1	0	—	—	0	—	—	8	1.97	2.60	8	1.07	4.06
+2	0	—	—	0	—	—	38	2.73	1.79	42	2.33	2.23
+3	0	—	—	0	—	—	53	2.87	1.89	56	2.76	1.70
+4	0	—	—	0	—	—	49	3.04	1.49	48	2.94	1.85
+5	0	—	—	0	—	—	46	3.27	1.48	40	3.16	1.53
+6	0	—	—	0	—	—	36	3.59	1.55	33	3.05	1.19
+7	0	—	—	0	—	—	26	3.57	1.04	25	3.02	1.34
+8	0	—	—	0	—	—	23	2.89	1.54	20	2.99	1.35
+9	0	—	—	0	—	—	20	2.90	1.48	14	3.26	1.07
+10	0	—	—	0	—	—	14	2.85	1.69	11	3.39	0.99

Source: See Table 17-5.

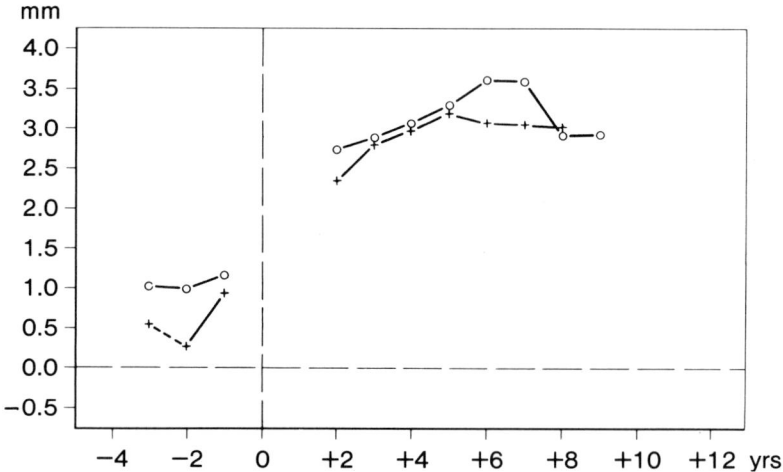

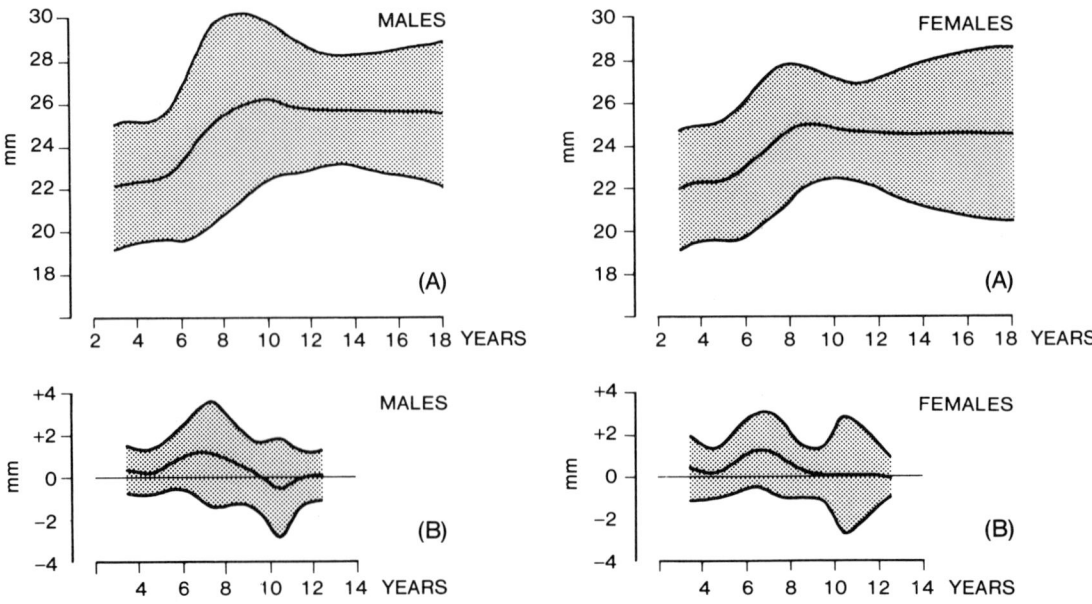

Figs. 17-6A and B   Distances between the mandibular canines (Mean ± 2 S.D.): (A) absolute values at various ages; (B) annual increments. (Derived from: Moorrees, C.F.A. The dentition of the growing child. Cambridge: Harvard University Press, 1979.)

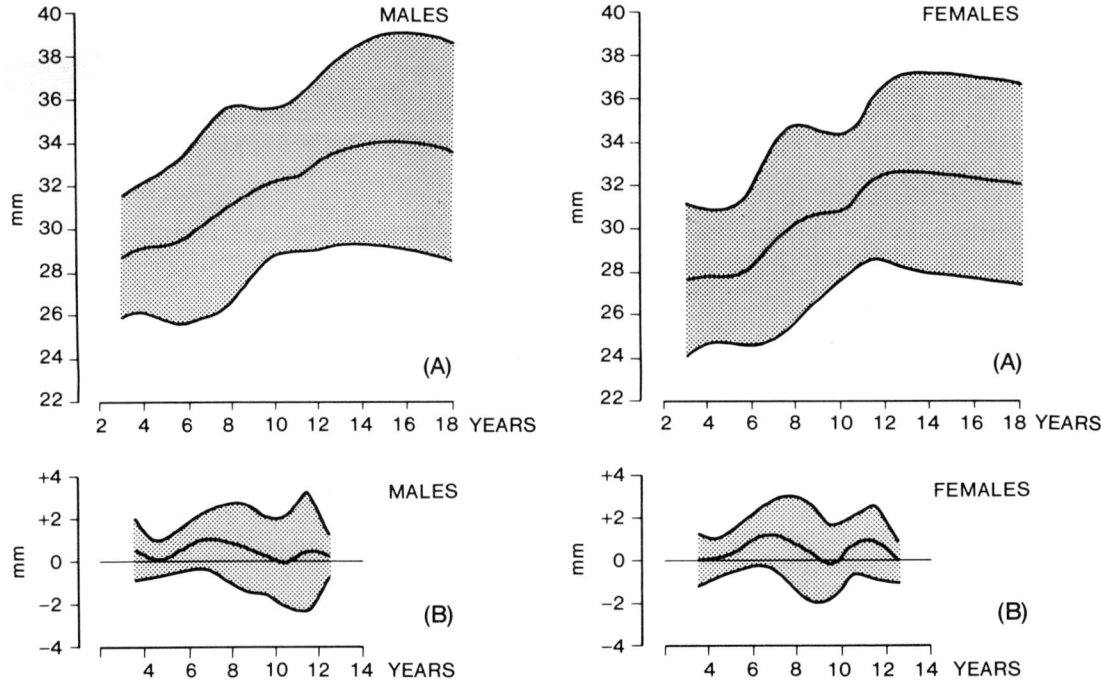

Figs. 17-7A and B   Distances between the maxillary canines (Mean ± 2 S.D.): (A) absolute values at various ages; (B) annual increments. (Source: see Figs. 17-6A and B.)

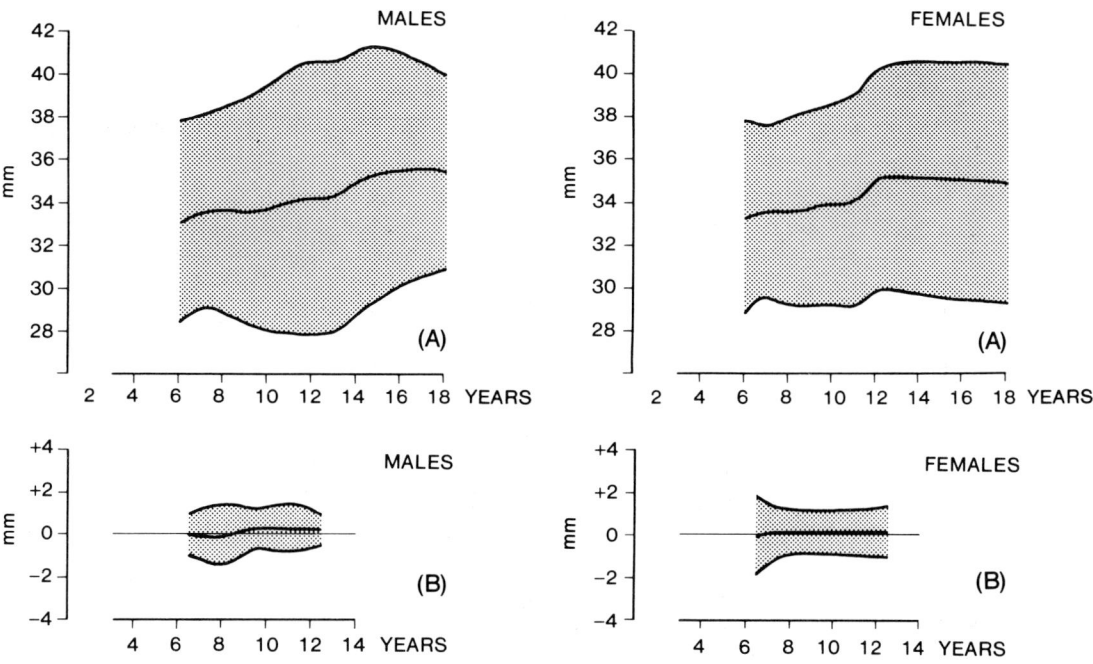

Figs. 17-8A and B Distances between the mandibular first permanent molars (Mean ± 2 S.D.): (A) absolute values at various ages; (B) annual increments. (Source see Figs. 17-6A and B.)

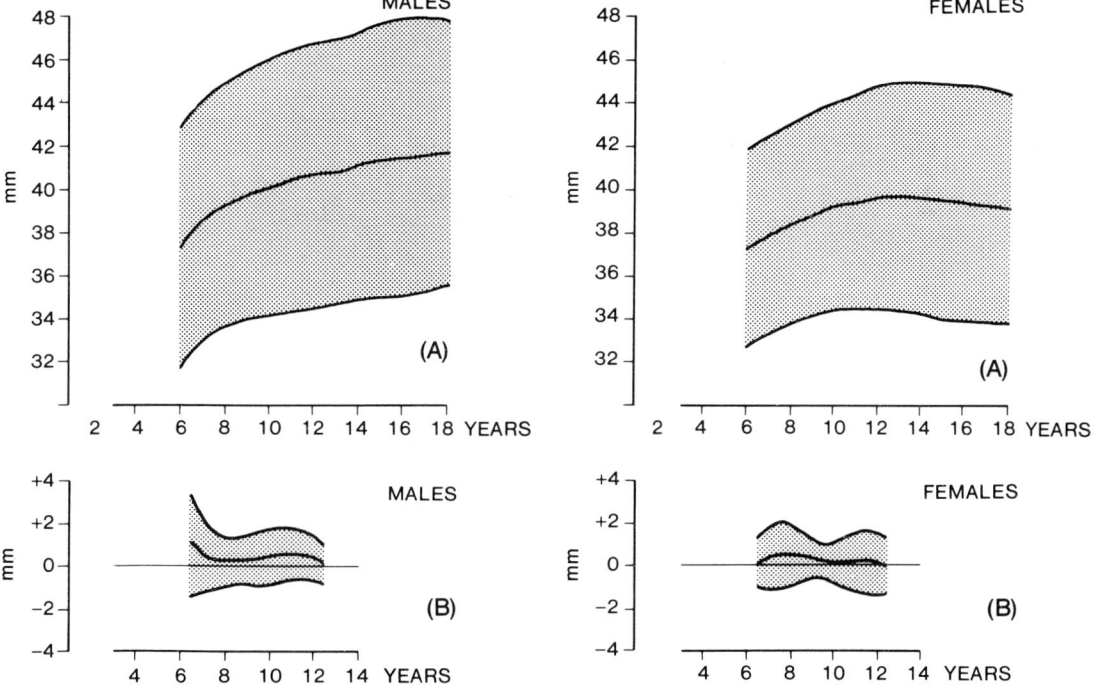

Figs. 17-9A and B Distances between the maxillary first permanent molars (Mean ± 2 S.D.): (A) absolute values at various ages; (B) annual increments. (Source: see Figs. 17-6A and B.)

Table 17-18 Emergence sequences for children from Oregon

Maxilla sequence* for girls	No. of subjects**	Mandible sequence for girls	No. of subjects	Maxilla sequence for boys	No. of subjects	Mandible sequence for boys	No. of subjects
2-3-5-4-6-1-7	12	1-3-4-5-6-2-7	21	2-3-6-4-5-1-7	9	1-3-4-5-6-2-7	9
2-3-6-4-5-1-7	9	1-3-4-5-7-2-6	9	2-3-4-4-5-1-6	4	1-3-4-5-7-2-6	6
2-3-4-5-6-1-7	9	2-3-4-5-6-1-7	6	1-3-4-6-5-2-7	4	1-2-3-4-5-1-6	4
1-3-5-4-6-2-7	7	1-2-3-4-5-1-6	5	2-3-5-4-6-1-7	4	1-3-6-4-5-2-7	4
2-3-4-4-5-1-6	5	1-3-5-4-6-2-7	5	2-3-4-5-6-1-7	3	2-3-4-5-6-1-7	4
2-3-4-5-7-1-6	5	2-3-5-4-6-1-7	5	2-3-5-4-4-1-6	3	2-3-4-5-7-1-6	4
2-3-5-4-7-1-6	5	2-3-4-5-7-1-6	4	2-3-5-4-6-1-6	3	1-2-4-5-6-3-7	2
1-2-5-3-4-1-6	4	1-3-4-4-5-2-6	3	2-3-6-4-7-1-5	3	1-3-4-4-5-2-6	2
2-3-4-4-4-1-5	4	1-3-4-6-5-2-7	3	1-2-5-3-4-1-6	2	1-3-5-4-7-2-6	2
2-3-5-6-4-1-7	4	1-2-3-4-5-1-4	2	2-3-4-4-6-1-5	2	2-3-4-4-5-1-6	2
2-3-5-4-5-1-6	3	1-2-3-4-5-2-6	2	2-3-4-5-5-1-6	2		
2-3-7-5-4-1-6	3	1-2-3-4-6-1-5	2	2-3-4-5-6-1-6	2		
1-3-6-4-5-2-7	2	1-2-5-3-4-1-6	2	2-3-4-5-7-1-6	2		
2-3-5-4-4-1-6	2	1-3-4-6-7-2-5	2	2-3-5-4-5-1-6	2		
2-3-6-4-7-1-5	2	2-2-3-4-6-1-5	2	2-3-5-4-7-1-6	2		
2-3-7-4-5-1-6	2						
Unique***	27	Unique	24	Unique	20	Unique	30
Total	105	Total	97	Total	67	Total	69

Derived from Savara, B.S., Steen, J.C.: Timing and sequence of eruption of permanent teeth in a longitudinal sample of children from Oregon. J. Amer. Dent. Assn. 97(1978):209.

*Sequence: central incisor, lateral incisor, canine, first premolar, second premolar, first molar, and second molar.
**Includes only dentitions with all seven teeth present in each quadrant.
***Sequences that occurred only once in the group.

Emergence Sequences

The data on emergence sequences (Table 17-18) are based on investigations in the United States and show a marked variation in emergence sequences, particularly of the canines and premolars. In Table 17-18 the emergence sequence is indicated with Arabic numerals on each line of the emergence sequence. In the indication of the emergence sequences, the order of teeth is I1, I2, C P1, P2, M1, M2. The first number in an emergence sequence represents the order of emergence of the central incisor among the seven permanent teeth studied. The second number in the sequence represents the order of emergence of the lateral incisor; the third number in the sequence represents the order of emergence of the canine, etc. Thus, an emergence sequence of, for example, 2-3-5-4-6-1-7 means that the first emerging tooth was the M1, the second the I1, the third the I2, the fourth the P1, the fifth the C, the sixth the P2, and the seventh the M2.[77] An emergence sequence such as 2-3-5-4-6-1-6 means that the P2 and M2 emerged simultaneously (i.e., within 3 months of each other) as the last two teeth in the series.

Numerical and Graphical Information

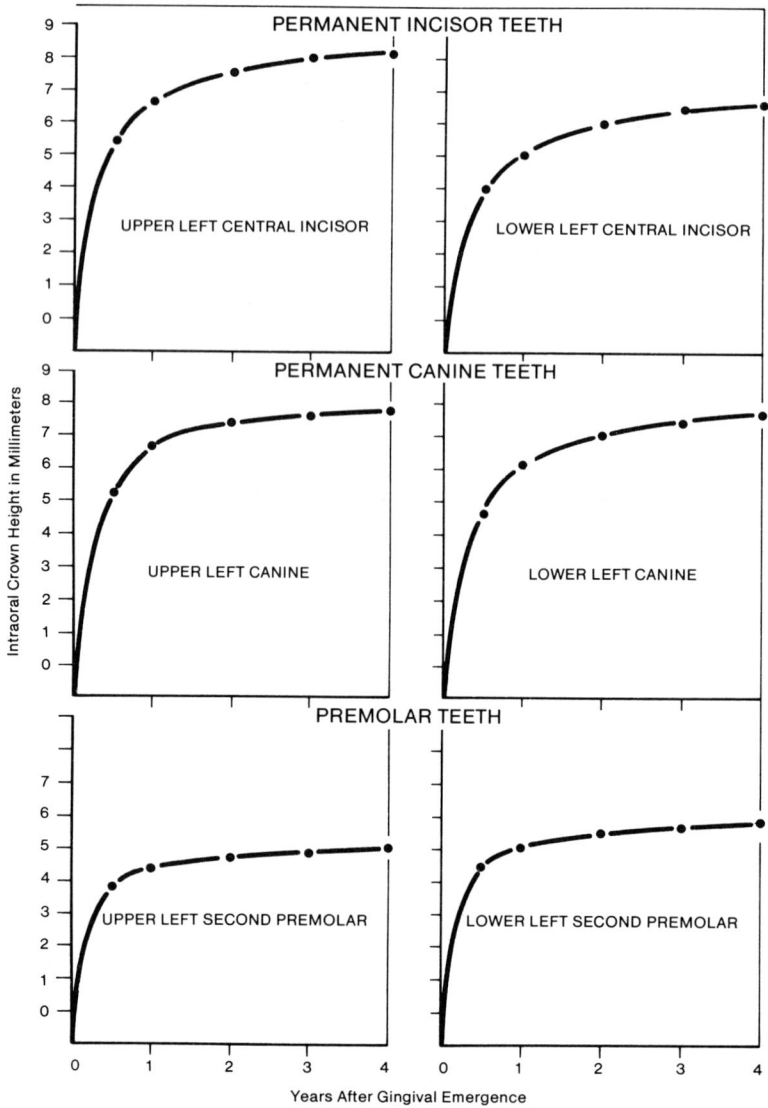

Fig. 17-10 Mean trends of increase in intraoral height for six permanent teeth. (Derived from Giles, N.B.; Knott, V.B.; and Meredith, H.V. Increase in intraoral height of selected permanent teeth during the quadrennium following gingival emergence. Angle Orthod. 33(1963):195.)

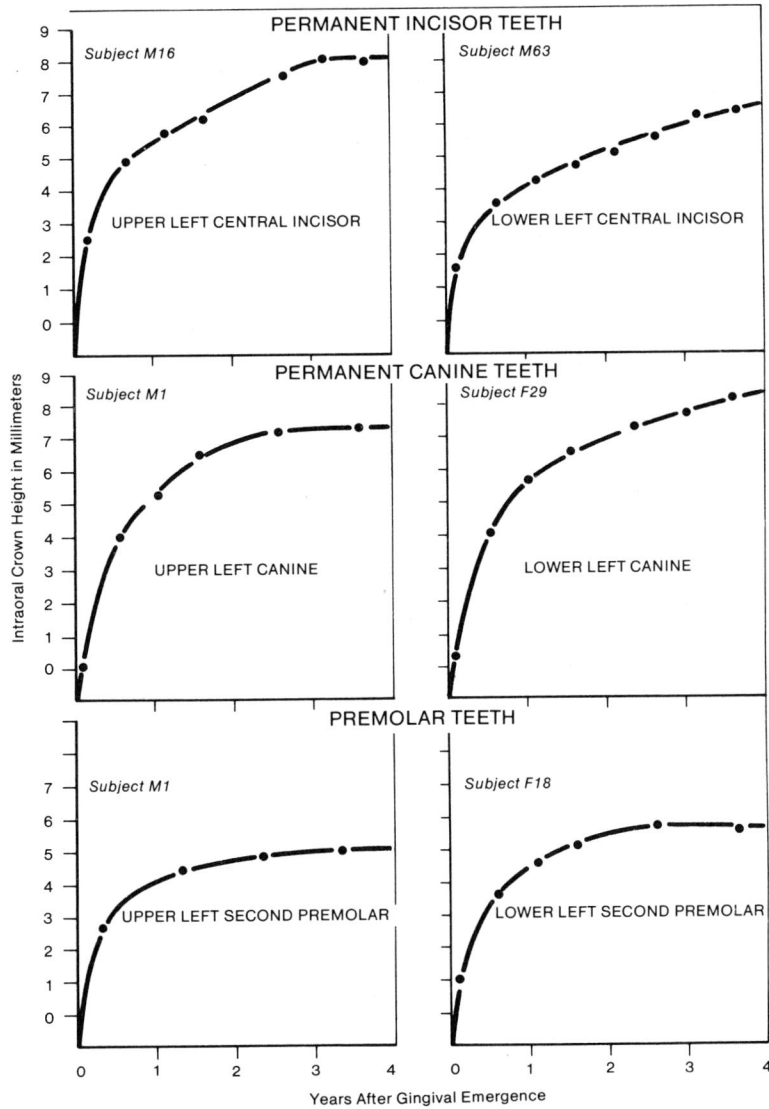

Fig. 17-11 Individual curves of intraoral tooth height. For each of six permanent teeth the curve shown is the one exhibiting minimum curvature in the triennium following gingival emergence. (Source: see Fig. 17-10.)

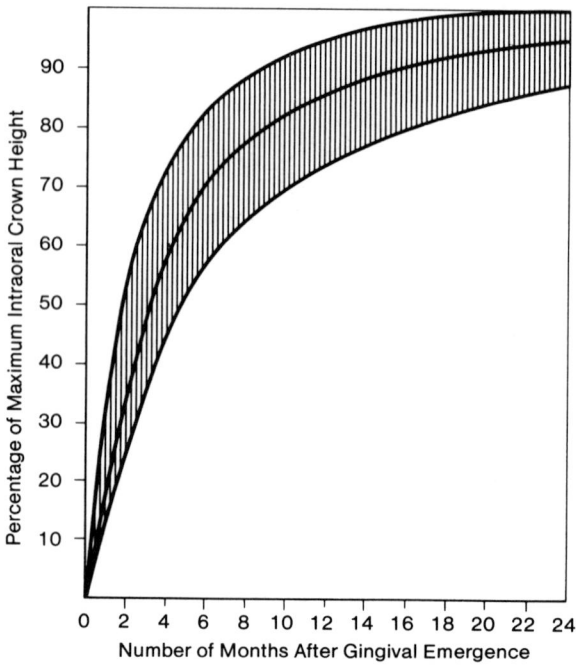

Fig. 17-12 Generalized reference chart depicting times children may take in erupting different percentages of maximum intraoral height of permanent incisor, canine, and premolar teeth. The horizontal width through the striped band gives on every level the time limits for approximately 80% of the children. (Source: see Fig. 17-10.)

Table 17-19 Occurrence of agenesis of teeth—percentages of observed agenesis for permanent teeth

	Boys (n = 4438)	Girls (n = 4256)	Boys and girls (n = 8694)
−5	4.21	4.53	4.37
+5	1.26	2.20	1.72
+2	1.19	2.18	1.67
−1	0.33	0.58	0.46
−2	0.33	0.56	0.44
−7	0.22	0.39	0.31
+4	0.20	0.21	0.20
+3	0.15	0.09	0.12
+6	0.09	0.16	0.12
+7	0.06	0.18	0.12
−4	0.11	0.11	0.11
−6	0.04	0.02	0.03
−3	0.02	0.04	0.03
+1	—	—	—

Based on Bachmann, H. Die Häufigkeit von Nichtanlagen bleibender Zähne (ausgenommen der Weisheitszähne). Ergebnis der Auswertung von 8694 Orthopantogrammen 9-10 jähriger Schulkinder aus Zürich. *Med. Diss. Zürich,* 1974.

Table 17-20 Occurrence of various jaw relations—comparison of past and present studies

Investigator	Location	Sample	Age	Number	Total malocclusion %	Normal %	Class I %	Class II %	Class III %
Angle (1907)	St. Louis	"Several thousand malocclusions"	Not given	1,000	100	—	69	26	4
Chiavaro (1913)	Not given	—	3–6 yrs	1,000	29	71	22	4	2
Thielemann (1922)	Leipzig	"Small children"	preschool	Not given	49	51	42	4	2
Korkhaus (1927)	Bonn	School children	6 yrs	643	43	Not given	77	16	6
			14 yrs	568	55	Not given	75	25	1
Hill, Blayney, Wolf (1959)	Evanston and Oak Park, Ill.	School children	6–8 yrs	4,251	30	69	20	9	1
			12–14 yrs	4,137	49	50	34	14	1
Emrich, Brodie, Blayney (1963)	Evanston and Oak Park, Ill.	School children	6–8 yrs	11,036	31	69	18	11	1
			12–14 yrs	14,951	45	53	30	15	1

Derived from Emrich, R.E., Brodie, A.G., and Blayney, J.R. Prevalence of Class I, Class II, and Class III malocclusions (Angle) in an urban population. An epidemiological study. J.Dent.Res. 44(1965):947.

Numerical and Graphical Information

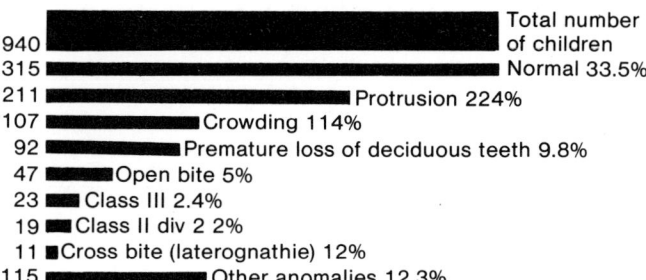

Fig. 17-13 Distribution of orthodontic anomalies in 940 school children selected from 30 schools (each 15th child). The sample may be considered as representative for the whole population of the city of Groningen, The Netherlands. Class II/1 malocclusion is indicated as "Protrusion." (Derived from Bijlstra, K.G. Frequency of dentofacial anomalies in school children and some aetiologic factors. Trans. Eur. Orthod. Soc. 231, 1958.)

Chapter 18

Concluding Remarks

The development of the dentition in the human being is a complex process and depends on many variables, which by no means always combine harmoniously. The teeth may deviate in number, size, shape, and position. The same holds true for the size, shape, and position of the bony structures in which the dentition is housed and for the changes that take place in the bony structures during growth. The role played by the soft tissues, particularly of the tongue and the lips and cheeks may vary significantly. The same holds true for the way in which the different functions of the orofacial region may be exerted. Taking all these factors into consideration, it is not surprising to note that the development of the human dentition rather seldom proceeds harmoniously and in an optimum way, and therefore an ideal end result is rarely achieved.

It is not simple to determine, in a specific example of a developing dentition, whether the situation at hand is normal or abnormal. The same applies even more to arriving at an adequate decision regarding the desirability of interfering with the natural development and implementing some therapy and, if so, when and how.

Without further explanation, it will be clear that to arrive at a good decision on the subjects mentioned above, an adequate knowledge of normal and abnormal development of the dentition is a first requisite. It is hoped that this book may have served as a worthwhile contribution in this respect.

References

1. Angle, E.H. 1899. Classification of malocclusion. *Dental Cosmos* 41: 248-64, 350-57.
2. Angle, E.H. 1907. *Treatment of malocclusion of the teeth* (7th ed.). Philadelphia: S.S. White.
3. Bachmann, H. 1974. *Die Häufigkeit von Nichtanlagen bleibender Zähne (ausgenommen der Weisheitszähne). Ergebnis der Auswertung von 8694 Orthopantogrammen 9-10 jähriger Schulkinder aus Zürich.* Med. Diss. Zürich.
4. *Bakker, P.J.M.R.; Wassenberg, H.J.W.; and van der Linden, F.P.G.M. 1979. Veränderungen im unteren Schneidezahnbereich im Zusammenhang mit dem Wechsel der seitlichen Unterkieferzähne. *Inf. Orthod. Kieferorthop.* 11:199-212.
5. *Bakker, P.J.M.R.; Wassenberg, H.J.W.; and van der Linden, F.P.G.M. 1979. Wechsel der oberen Schneidezähne. *Inf. Orthod. Kieferorthop.* 11:239-70.
6. *Bakker, P.J.M.R.; Wassenberg, H.J.W.; and van der Linden, F.P.G.M. 1979. Wechsel der unteren Schneidezähne. *Inf. Orthod. Kieferorthop.* 11:144-68.
7. Baume, L.J. 1950. Physiological tooth migration and its significance for the development of occlusion. I. The biogenetic course of the deciduous dentition. *J. Dent. Res.* 29: 123-32.
8. Baume, L.J. 1950. Physiological tooth migration and its significance for the development of occlusion. II. The biogenesis of the accessional dentition. *J. Dent. Res.* 29: 331-37.
9. Baume, L.J. 1950. Physiological tooth migration and its significance for the development of occlusion. III. The biogenesis of the successional dentition. *J. Dent. Res.* 29: 338-48.

*References 4, 5, 6, 105, 109, 110, 112, 113 and 114 have been published also in English in a monograph listed as reference 104.

10. Berendsen, W.J.H. 1978. Personal communication.
11. Berkovitz, B.K.B. 1976. Theories of tooth eruption. In *The eruption and occlusion of teeth,* eds. D.F.G. Poole and M.V. Stack, Colston Papers No. 27. Boston: Butterworths.
12. Bijlstra, K.G. 1958. Frequency of dentofacial anomalies in school children and some aetiologic factors. *Trans. Eur. Orthod. Soc.* 231-36.
13. Björk, A. 1947. *The face in profile.* Svensk. Trandläk. Tidsk. 40, suppl. 5B.
14. Björk, A. 1953. Variability and age changes in overjet and overbite. *Amer. J. Orthod.* 39: 779-801.
15. Bodegom, J.C. 1969. *Experiments on tooth eruption in miniature pigs.* Doctoral thesis, University of Nymegen.
16. Bolton, W.A. 1958. Disharmony in tooth size and its relation to the analysis of malocclusion. *Angle Orthod.* 38: 113-30.
17. Bolton, W.A. 1962. The clinical application of a tooth size analysis. *Amer. J. Orthod.* 48: 504-29.
18. Bonnar, E.M.E. 1956. Aspects of the transition from deciduous to permanent dentition. *Dent. Pract., Dent. Rec.* (Bristol) 7: 42-54.
19. Brauer, J.E. 1941. A report of 113 early or premature extractions of primary molars and the incidence of closure of space. *J. Dent. Child.* 8: 222-24.
20. Breakspear, E.K. 1961. Further observations on early loss of deciduous molars. *Dent. Pract., Dent. Rec.* (Bristol) 11: 233-52.
21. Broadbent, B.H. 1937. The face of the normal child. *Angle Orthod.* 7: 183-208.
22. Broadbent, B.H. 1941. Ontogenic development of occlusion. *Angle Orthod.* 11: 223-41.
23. Clinch, L.M. 1934. Variations in the

References

mutual relationship of the maxillary and mandibular gum pads in the new born child. *Int. J. Orthod.* 20: 359-72.

24. Clinch, L.M. 1951. An analysis of serial models between three and eight years of age. *Dent. Rec.* 71: 61-72.
25. Clinch, L.M. 1959. A longitudinal study of the results of premature loss of deciduous teeth between 3-4 and 13-14 years of age. *Dent. Pract., Dent. Rec. (Bristol)* 9: 109-28.
26. Davey, K.W. 1966. Effect of premature loss of deciduous molars on the antero-posterior position of maxillary first permanent molars and other maxillary teeth. *J. Can. Dent. Assn.* 32: 406-16.
27. De Boer, M. 1970. *Aspekten van de gebitsontwikkeling bij kinderen tussen vijf en tien jaar.* Doctoral thesis. University of Utrecht.
28. Demirjian, A.; Goldstein, H.; and Tanner, J.M. 1973. A new system of dental age assessment. *Hum. Biol.* 45: 211-27.
29. Dempster, W.T.; Adams, W.J.; and Duddles, R.A. 1963. Arrangement in the jaws of the roots of the teeth. *J. Amer. Dent. Assn.* 67: 779-97.
30. Emrich, R.E.; Brodie, A.G.; and Blayney, J.R. 1965. Prevalence of Class I, Class II, and Class III malocclusions (Angle) in an urban population. An epidemiological study. *J. Dent. Res.* 44: 947-53.
31. Falck, F., and Fränkel, R. 1973. Die labiale Alveolenwand unter dem Einfluss des durchbrechenden Schneidezahnes. *Fortschr. Kieferorthop.* 34: 37-47.
32. Fanning, E.A. 1958. A longitudinal study of tooth calcification and root resorption. *J. Dent. Res.* 73: 4.
33. Fanning, E.A. 1961. A longitudinal study of tooth formation and root resorption. *New Zeal. Dent. J.* 57: 202-217.
34. Fanning, E.A. 1962. Effect of extraction of deciduous molars on the formation and eruption of their successors. *Angle Orthod.* 32: 44-53.
35. Fleming, H.B. 1961. An investigation of the vertical overbite during the eruption of the permanent dentition. *Angle Orthod.* 31: 53-62.
36. Fletcher, G.G.T. 1975. The retroclined upper incisor. *Brit. J. Orthod.* 2: 207-16.
37. Fränkel, R., and Falck, F. 1967. Zahndurchbruch und Vererbung beim Deckbiss. *Fortschr. Kieferorthop.* 28: 175-82.
38. Friel, S. 1954. The development of ideal occlusion of the gum pads and the teeth. *Amer. J. Orthod.* 40: 196-227.
39. Giles, N.B.; Knott, V.B.; and Meredith, H.V. 1963. Increase in intraoral height of selected permanent teeth during the quadrennium following gingival emergence. *Angle Orthod.* 33: 195-206.
40. Helm, S., and Siersbaek-Nielsen, S. 1973. Crowding in the permanent dentition after early loss of deciduous molars or canines. *Trans. Eur. Orthod. Soc.* 137-49.
41. Hoffding, J., and Kisling, E. 1979. Premature loss of primary teeth. I. Its overall effect on occlusion and space in the permanent dentition. *J. Dent. Child.* 45: 279-83.
42. Hoffding, J., and Kisling, E. 1979. Premature loss of primary teeth. II. The specific effect on occlusion and space in the permanent dentition. *J. Dent. Child.* 45: 284-87.
43. Hunter, J. 1771. *The natural history of the human teeth; explaining their structure, use, formation, growth and diseases.* London: J. Johnson.
44. Hurme, V.O. 1949. Ranges of normalcy in the eruption of permanent teeth. *J. Dent. Child.* 16: 11-15.
45. Jacobsson, S.O. 1965. Diastema mediale. En longitudinell undersökning. *Odont. Tidskr.* 73: 127-48.
46. Knott, V.B., and Meredith, M.V. 1966. Statistics on eruption of the permanent dentition from serial data from North American white children. *Angle Orthod.* 36: 68-79.
47. Kolf, J. 1976. Le syndrome hypertonique antérieur ou propos sur la Classe II, div. 2. *Rev. d'Orthop. Dento-Fac.* 10: 149-62.
48. Korf, S.R. 1965. The eruption of permanent central incisors following premature loss of their antecedents. *J. Dent. Child.* 32: 39-44.
49. Kraus, B.S., and Jordan, R.E. 1965. *The human dentition before birth.* Philadelphia: Lea & Febiger.
50. Kraus, B.S.; Jordan, R.E.; and Abrams, L. 1969. *Dental anatomy and occlusion.* Baltimore: Williams & Wilkins.

51. Lande, M.J. 1952. Growth behavior of the human bony facial profile as revealed by serial cephalometric roentgenology. *Angle Orthod.* 22: 78-90.
52. Lear, C.S.C.; Flanagan, J.B.; and Moorrees, C.F.A. 1965. The frequency of deglutition in man. *Arch. Oral. Biol.* 10: 83-99.
53. Linder—Aronson, S. 1960. The effect of premature loss of deciduous teeth. A biometric study in 14- and 15-year olds. *Acta Odont. Scand.* 18: 101-22.
54. Lo, R.T., and Moyers, R.E. 1953. Studies in the etiology and prevention of malocclusion. I. The sequence of eruption of the permanent dentition. *Amer. J. Orthod.* 39: 460-67.
55. Logan, W.H.G., and Kronfeld, R. 1933. Development of the human jaws and surrounding structures from birth to the age of fifteen years. *J. Amer. Dent. Assn.* 20: 379-427.
56. Lundström, A. 1955. The significance of early loss of deciduous teeth in the etiology of malocclusion. *Amer. J. Orthod.* 41: 819-26.
57. Lysell, L.; Magnusson, B.; and Thilander, B. 1962. Time and order of eruption of the primary teeth. *Odont. Revy* 13: 217-34.
58. Magnusson, T.E. 1979. The effect of premature loss of deciduous teeth on the spacing of the permanent dentition *Eur. J. Orthod.* 1: 243-49.
59. Meyer, W. 1932. *Lehrbuch der normalen Histologie und Entwicklungsgeschichte der Zähne des Menschen.* München: J.F. Lehrmanns Verlag.
60. Mills, J.R.E. 1973. The problem of overbite in Class II, division 2 malocclusion. *Brit. J. Orthod.* 1: 34-48.
61. Moore, A.W. 1956. The mechanism of adjustment to wear and accident in the dentition and periodontium. *Angle Orthod.* 26: 50-58.
62. Moore, A.W. 1960. Personal communication.
63. Moorrees, C.F.A. 1959: *The dentition of the growing child: a longitudinal study of dental development between 3 and 18 years of age.* Cambridge: Harvard University Press.
64. Moorrees, C.F.A. 1965. Normal variation in dental development determined with reference to tooth eruption status. *J. Dent. Res.* 44: 161-73.
65. Moorrees, C.F.A., and Chadha, J.M. 1962. Crown diameters of corresponding tooth groups in the deciduous and permanent dentition. *J. Dent. Res.* 41: 466-70.
66. Moorrees, C.F.A., and Chadha, J.M. 1965. Available space for the incisors during dental development. *Angle Orthod.* 35: 12-22.
67. Moorrees, C.F.A.; Fanning, E.A.; Grön, A.M.; and Lebret, L. 1962. The timing of orthodontic treatment in relation to tooth formation. *Trans. Eur. Orthod. Soc.* 87-101.
68. Moorrees, C.F.A.; Fanning, E.A.; and Hunt, Jr., E.E. 1963. Age variation of formation stages for ten permanent teeth. *J. Dent. Res.* 42: 1490-1502.
69. Moorrees, C.F.A., and Kent, R.L. 1977. Patterns of dental maturation. In *The biology of occlusal development,* ed. J.A. McNamara, Jr., Monograph No. 7, Craniofacial growth series, Center for Human Growth and Development. Ann Arbor: The University of Michigan, pp. 25-41.
70. Moorrees, C.F.A., and Reeds, R.B. 1964. Correlations among crown diameters of human teeth. *Arch. Oral Biol.* 9: 685-97.
71. Moyers, R.E. 1973. *Handbook of orthodontics* (3rd ed.). Chicago: Year Book Med. Publ.
72. Moyers, R.E.; van der Linden, F.P.G.M.; Riolo, M.L.; and McNamara, Jr., J.A. 1976. *Standards of human occlusal development.* Monograph No. 5, Craniofacial growth series, Center for Human Growth and Development. Ann Arbor: The University of Michigan.
73. Nanda, R.S. 1960. Eruption of human teeth. *Amer. J. Orthod.* 46: 363-78.
74. Neff, C.W. 1964. *Frequency of deglutition of tongue thrusters compared to a population of normal swallowers.* M.S.D. thesis, University of Washington, Seattle.
75. Nicol, W.A. 1963. The lower lip and the upper incisor teeth in Angle's Class II, division 2 malocclusion. *Dent. Pract., Dent. Rec.* (Bristol) 14: 179-82.
76. Nolla, C. 1960. Development of the permanent teeth. *J. Dent. Child.* 27: 254-266.
77. Northway, W.M. 1977. *Anteroposterior*

References

arch dimension changes in French-Canadian children: a study of the effects of dental caries and premature extractions. M. Sc. thesis, University of Montreal.

78. Owen, D. 1971. The incidence and nature of space closure following the premature extraction of deciduous teeth. A literature survey. *Amer. J. Orthod.* 59: 37-49.
79. Posen, A.L. 1972. The influence of maximum perioral and tongue forces on the incisor teeth. *Angle Orthod.* 42: 285-309.
80. Prahl-Andersen, B., and Berendsen, W.J.H. 1979. Enige gevolgen van vroegtijdig verlies van tweede melkmolaren in de onderkaak. *Ned. Tijdschr. Tandhk.* 86: 89-92.
81. Prahl-Andersen, B.; Kowalski, C.W.; and Heydendael, P.H.J., eds. 1979. *A mixed-longitudinal, interdisciplinary study of growth and development.* New York: Academic Press.
82. Prahl-Andersen, B., and van der Linden, F.P.G.M. 1972. The estimation of dental age. *Trans. Eur. Orthod. Soc.* 535-41.
83. Richardson, M.E. 1965. The relationship between the relative amount of space present in the deciduous dental arch and the rate and degree of space closure subsequent to extraction of a deciduous molar. *Dent. Pract., Dent. Rec.* (Bristol) 16: 111-18.
84. Robinow, M.; Richards, T.W.; and Anderson, M. 1942. The eruption of deciduous teeth. *Growth* 6: 127-33.
85. Rönnerman, A. 1965. Early extraction of deciduous molars and canines. *Trans. Eur. Orthod. Soc.* 153-68.
86. Rönnerman, A. 1977. The effect of early loss of primary molars on tooth eruption and space conditions. A longitudinal study. *Acta Odont. Scand.* 35:229-39.
87. Savara, B.S., and Steen, J.C. 1978. Timing and sequence of eruption of permanent teeth in a longitudinal sample of children from Oregon. *J. Amer. Dent. Assn.* 97: 209-14.
88. Schour, I. 1929. Early human tooth development with special reference to the relationship between the dental lamina and the lip-furrow band. *J. Dent. Res.* 9: 699-717.
89. Schwarz, A.M. 1951. *Lehrgang der Gebissregelung* (2nd ed.). Wien-Innsbruck: Urban und Schwarzenberg.
90. Seipel, C.M. 1948. Prevention of malocclusion. *Trans. Eur. Orthod. Soc.* 203-13.
91. Shumaker, D.B., and El Hadary, M.S. 1960. Roentgenographic study of eruption. *J. Amer. Dent. Assn.* 61: 535-41.
92. Sicher, H. 1960. *Oral Anatomy* (3rd ed.), St. Louis: C.V. Mosby.
93. Sillman, J.H. 1938. Relationship of maxillary and mandibular gum pads in the newborn infant. *Amer. J. Orthod.* 24: 409-24.
94. Sillman, J. H. 1964. Dimensional changes of the dental arches: longitudinal study from birth to 25 years. *Amer. J. Orthod.* 50: 824-42.
95. Smith, R.J., and Rapp, R. 1980. A cephalometric study of the developmental relationship between primary and permanent maxillary central incisor teeth. *J. Dent. Child.* 36: 36-41.
96. Stöckli, P.W. 1976. Postnataler Wachstumsverlauf, Kieferwachstum und Entwicklung der Dentition. In *Zahnmedizin bei Kindern und Jugendlichen,* ed. R.P. Hotz. Stuttgart: George Thieme Verlag, pp. 27-87.
97. Streeter, G.L. 1948. Developmental horizons in human embryos. *Contrib. Embryol. Carnegie* 32 (211):133-203, 31: 27.
98. Sturdivant, J.E.; Knott, V.B.; and Meredith, H.V. 1962. Interrelations from serial data for eruption of the permanent dentition. *Angle Orthod.* 32: 1-13.
99. Ungar, A.L. 1938. Incidence and effects of premature loss of deciduous teeth. *Int. J. Orthod.* 24: 613-21.
100. Van Alstine, Jr., W.L., and Moyers, R.E. 1978. Personal Communication.
101. van der Linden, F.P.G.M. 1970. Interrelated factors in the morphogenesis of teeth, the development of the dentition and craniofacial growth. *Schweiz. Monatschr. Zahnheilk.* 80: 518-26.
102. van der Linden, F.P.G.M. 1975. Zwei Varianten der Klasse II/1. *Fortschr. Kieferorthop.* 36: 51-72.
103. van der Linden, F.P.G.M. 1978. Changes in the position of posterior teeth in relation to ruga points. *Amer. J. Orthod.* 74: 142-61.

104. van der Linden, F.P.G.M., ed. 1982. *Transition of the human dentition.* Monograph No. 13, Craniofacial growth series, Center for Human Growth and Development. Ann Arbor: The University of Michigan.
105. *van der Linden, F.P.G.M.; Bakker, P.J.M.R.; and Wassenberg, H.J.W. 1979. Anmerkungen bezüglich der Entwicklung der Dentition und der Durchführung der kieferorthopädischen Therapie. *Inf. Orthod. Kieferorthop.* 11: 319-23.
106. van der Linden, F.P.G.M.; Boersma, H.; and Prahl-Andersen, B. 1979. Development of the dentition. In *A mixed-longitudinal interdisciplinary study of growth and development,* eds. B. Prahl-Andersen, C.J. Kowalski, and P.H.J. Heydendael. New York: Academic Press, pp. 521-36.
107. van der Linden, F.P.G.M. and Duterloo, H.S. 1976. *Development of the human dentition. An atlas.* Hagerstown, Md. Harper & Row.
108. van der Linden, F.P.G.M.; McNamara, Jr., J.A.; and Burdi, A.R. 1972. Tooth size and position before birth. *J. Dent. Res.* 51: 71-74.
109. *van der Linden, F.P.G.M.; Wassenberg, H.J.W.; and Bakker, P.J.M.R. 1979. Allgemeine Aspekte der Entwicklung des Gebisses. *Inf. Orthod. Kieferorthop.* 11: 131-33.
110. *van der Linden, F.P.G.M.; Wassenberg, H.J.W.; and Bakker, P.J.M.R. 1979. Der Übergangsprozess im Rückblick. *Inf. Orthod. Kieferorthop.* 11: 325-30.
111. Van Hillegondsberg, A.J. 1959. *Over de betekenis van enkele postnatale factoren voor het ontstaan van dentomaxillaire afwijkingen in het temporare gebit.* Doctoral thesis, University of Utrecht.
112. *Wassenberg, H.J.W.; Bakker, P.J.M.R.; and van der Linden, F.P.G.M. 1979. Änderungen im oberen Schneidezahnbereich im Zusammenhang mit dem Wechsel der seitlichen Oberkieferzähne. *Inf. Orthod. Kieferorthop.* 11: 305-18.
113. *Wassenberg, H.J.W.; Bakker, P.J.M.R.; and van der Linden, F.P.G.M. 1979. Wechsel der seitlichen Oberkieferzähne. *Inf. Orthod. Kieferorthop.* 11: 271-304.
114. *Wassenberg, H.J.W.; Bakker, P.J.M.R.; and van der Linden, F.P.G.M. 1979. Wechsel der seitlichen Unterkieferzähne. *Inf. Orthod. Kieferorthop.* 11: 169-98.

*See note on page 203.

Index

A

Abnormal habits	115, *116*
thumb/finger sucking	115, *116, 117*
Abrams, L.	55
Adams, W.J.	56
Agenesis	72, *73*, 197
Anderson, M.	163
Angle, E.H.	81, 121
Angle classification	81
Ankylosis	72, 78, 79, 117
Arch, dental	
changes in dimensions	36, 59, 60, *61, 62, 64, 73,* 161, 172-183, 190, 191
dimension	161, 172-183
shape/form	29, *30, 44, 56*, 82, *85,* 89, 105
Arch length discrepancy (ALD)	71

B

Bachmann, H.	72, 197
Bakker, P.J.M.R.	37-39, 54, 165
Baume, L.J.	37, 65
Berendsen, W.J.H.	129, 131
Berkovitz, B.K.B.	41
Bijlstra, K.G.	9, 199
Björk, A.	60
Blayney, J.R.	198
Bodegom, J.C.	66
Boersma, H.	50, 163, 172-179
Bolton, W.A.	72
Bonnar, E.M.E.	65
Brauer, J.C.	130
Breakspear, E.K.	130, 131, 135
Broadbent, B.H.	38, 162
Brodie, A.G.	198
Brodie syndrome	124, *131*
Buccal musculature	42, 155, 160
Burdi, A.R.	17, 18, 22

C

Chadha, J.M.	39, 171
Class I malocclusion with Class II/2 symptoms	*102*, 103
Class I occlusion	79, 81
Class II/1 malocclusion	81-91, *83-86, 88, 90*, 139, 143
Class II/2 malocclusion	81, *94*, 93-103, 143
type A	93, *96*, 97
type B	93, *98*, 99
type C	93, *100*, 101
Class II occlusion	79
Class III malocclusion	81, 105-114, *106-108, 110, 112,* 143
Class II Subdivision	81, 121, *122*
Class III Subdivision	81, 121, *122*
Class III occlusion	79
Clinch, L.M.	23, 59, 130
Cone-funnel mechanism	26, 27, 35, 82, 117
Cross-bite	*122, 123*, 124, *126*
Crowding	68, 71, 79, 103, 129, 130, 133
before birth	21
in deciduous dentition	23
in mixed dentition	50
in permanent dentition	75

Index

Crown sizes 169
  of corresponding deciduous and permanent teeth   34, 38, 39, *48*, 50, 51, *52*
  of deciduous molars   29, 33, *34*, 50, 51
  differences in dimensions   50, 51
Curve of Spee   60

D

Davey, K.W.   131
De Boer, M.   130
Deciduous dentition
  complete   29, *30*
  development of   23, *24*, *25*, 27
Demirjian, A.   166, 167
Dempster, W.T.   55
Dental arch, *See* Arch
Dental lamina   11
Department of Orthodontics, University of Groningen School Study   9
Diastema(ta)
  central   36, *44*, 71
  in deciduous dentition   23, 29, *30*
  in mixed dentition   36, *43*, *46*, *48*, 65
  in permanent dentition   71
"Dished-in" profile   72, 98
Disto-occlusion   79
Double protrusion (D.P.)   72
Duddles, R.A.   55
Duterloo, H.S.   9, 27, 29, 33, 41, 46, 54

E

El Hadary, M.S.   66
Emergence   66
  deciduous teeth   23, *24*, *25*
  permanent teeth   33, *36*, 39, 41
  sequence of deciduous teeth   *24*, *25*
  sequence of permanent teeth   47, 192
  simultaneous   50, *52*
  times of deciduous teeth   53, 163
  times of permanent teeth   53, 131, 163, *164*
  variation in   50, 51, *52*, 163, *164*
Emrich, R.E.   198
Enamel,
  formation, *See* tooth/teeth morphogenesis
  hypocalcification   12
Endo-occlusion   124, *128*
"End-to-end" occlusion   91
Eruption process   36, 39, 41, 42, 65, *194-196*
Eversion   79
Exo-occlusion   124, *131*

F

Falck, F.   95
Fanning, E.A.   41, 66, 130, 162
First transitional period   33-42
Flanagan, J.B.   58
Fleming, H.B.   60
Fletcher, G.G.T.   95
"Forced bite"   109, 121, *123*, *125*
Forces of mastication   82
Fränkel, R.   95
Friel, S.   65
Function   155, 160

G

Giles, N.B.   39, 42, 66, 194-196
Goldstein, H.   166, 167
Grön, A.M.   41
Gubernacular canal   41, 51

H

Helm, S.   130, 131, 135
Heydendael, P.H.J.   9, 161, 165
Hoffding, J.   130
Horizontal overbite   79
Hunt, Jr., E.E.   162
Hunter, J.   46
Hurme, V.O.   50, 164

Index

I

Infraposition 72
Intertransitional period 38, 43-46

J

Jacobsson, S.O. 38
Jaw(s)
    growth, postnatal 23, *24, 25,* 33, 43, 54, 59, 60, *61,* 68, 69, 82, 155
    growth, prenatal *20,* 22
    transverse development 23, 59, 60, *61,* 82
Jordan, R.E. 13, 14, 17, 18, 55

K

Kent, R.L. 53, 170
Kisling, E. 130
Knott, V.G. 39, 42, 50, 66, 194-196
Kolf, J. 95
Korf, S.R. 131
Kowalski, C.W. 9, 161, 165
Kraus, B.S. 13, 14, 17, 18, 55
Kronfeld, R. 162

L

Labioinclination 76, 79
Labioposition 76, 79
Labioversion 79
Lande, M.J. 60
Lear, C.S.C. 58
Lebret, L. 41
Linder-Aronson, S. 131
Linguoinclination 76, 79
Linguoposition 76, 79
Linguoversion 79
Lip(s) 42, 43, 57, 58, 81, 89, 93-103, *96, 98, 100, 102,* 105, *110,* 114, 143, 155, *156,* 160
Lo, R.T. 47

Logan, W.H.G. 162
Lundström, A. 130
Lysell, L. 163

M

Magnusson, B. 131, 135, 163
Mandible,
    growth of, See jaw growth.
Maxilla,
    growth of, See jaw growth.
McNamara, Jr., J.A. 9, 17, 18, 22, 37, 59, 165, 169, 180-189
Meredith, H.V. 39, 42, 50, 66, 194-196
Mesiodens *72, 74*
Mesio-occlusion 79
Meyer, W. 162
Midline deviation 121, *123,* 133, *149,* 150, *151*
Mills, J.R.E. 95
Moore, A.W. 57, 124
Moorrees, C.F.A. 37, 39, 41, 53, 58, 59, 162, 165, 170, 171, 190, 191
Mouth breathing 155
Moyers, R.E. 9, 37, 47, 59, 66, 165, 169, 180-189

N

Nanda, R.S. 50
Nasal passage 155
Neff, C.W. 58
Neutro-occlusion 79
Nicol, W.A. 95
Nolla, C. 41, 66, 162
Northway, W.M. 130
Nymegen Growth Study 9

O

Occlusal plane 29, 60
Occlusion, establishment of dental 23, 27, 39, *48,* 51, 53, 60, 66

of deciduous dentition	29, *30*	Riolo, M.L.	9, 37, 59, 165, 169, 180-189
of mixed dentition	*44*	Robinow, M.	163
of permanent dentition	*56*	Rönnerman, A.	130, 131
Open bite	115-120, *119*		
Overbite	60, 79, *85, 86,* 89, *94, 96, 98, 100,* 133, 143, *151-153,* 188-189	**S**	
Overjet	60, 79, *85, 86,* 89, 133, 143, *151-153,* 186, 187	Sagittal overbite	79
		Savara, B.S.	50, 192
Owen, D.	131	Schour, I.	11
		Schwarz, A.M.	27
P		Second transitional period	38, 47-54
		Seipel, C.M.	131
Palatoinclincation	79	Shumaker, D.B.	66
Palatoposition	79	Sicher, H.	82
Palatoversion	79	Siersbaek-Nielsen, S.	131, 135
Permanent dentition	55-58	Sillman, J.H.	23, 59
Posen, A.L.	98	Smith, R.J.	40
Postnormal occlusion	79	Spacing	71, 134
Prahl-Andersen, B.	9, 50, 131, 161, 163, 166-168, 172-179	in deciduous dentition	23
		in mixed dentition	*36, 48,* 51
Premature loss of deciduous teeth	129-154	in permanent dentition	71
		Steen, J.C.	50, 192
of canines	*132, 134*	Stöckli, P.W.	162, 163
of incisors	*132, 134*	Stomion	93
of molars	*136-138, 140-142, 144-148*	Streeter, G.L.	21
Prenormal occlusion	79	Sturdivant, J.E.	50
Proclination	79	Subdivisions (Angle),	
Proposition	79	See Class II Subdivision	
Protrusion	79	See Class III Subdivision	
		Supraposition	72
		Suture, Intermaxillary	23, 82
R		Swallowing	58, 115, 155
		Symphysis, mandibular	82
Rapp, R.	40	Synchondrosis, mandibular	23
Reeds, R.B.	170		
Resorption of deciduous roots	*36, 40,* 41, 46, 50, *52,* 65, 129	**T**	
		Tanner, J.M.	166, 167
Retroinclination	79	Telescope bite	124, *127*
Retroposition	79	Terminal plane	33, *34, 52,* 65, 89
Retroversion	79	Thilander, B.	163
Retrusion	79	Tongue	42, 43, 57, 58, 114, 115, 155, *158,* 160
Reversed overjet	105, *108, 110*		
Richards, T.W.	163		
Richardson, M.E.	130	Tooth size discrepancy (TSD)	72, *75*

Index

Tooth/Teeth,
    angulation, See orientation/position
    arrangement before birth   17, 18, *20*, 22
    calcification   12, *13-19*, 39, 46, 66, 162
    color   12
    deviations in position   72
    formation   11, 12, 29, 38, 46, 66, 68, 72, 165, *166-168*
    impaction   78
    inclination, See orientation/position
    morphogenesis   11, 12, *13-19*
    orientation/position of deciduous   29, *30*, 33, *36*, 39, *40*, 43, *52*, 68
    orientation/position of permanent   *36*, *40*, 42, 46, *48*, 55, *56*, *58*, 68, 76, 77, *149*, *156*, *158*
    position prior to emergence   21, 29, *30*, 33, *36*, 38-40, *44*, 47-54, *48*
    shape deviations   72
    size deviations   72, *75*
    supernumerary   72, *74*
Transition,
    of incisors   33-42, *36*, *40*
    of posterior teeth   47-54, *48*
Trauma   78, 131

U

Ungar, A.L.   130
The University of Michigan Elementary and Secondary School of Study   9

V

Van Alstine, Jr., W.L.   66
van der Linden, F.P.G.M.   9, 17, 18, 22, 23, 27, 29, 33, 38, 39, 41, 46, 50, 54, 59, 88, 163, 165-169, 172-189
Van Hillegondsberg, A.J.   117
Vertical overbite   79

W

Wassenberg, H.J.W.   37-39, 54, 165